Grow Your Dermatology Practice

with a Nurse Practitioner or Physician Assistant

The Ultimate Guide to Hiring, Educating, and Integrating an NP or a PA

by Roger T. Moore, MD

Dermwise™

Grow Your Dermatology Practice with a Nurse Practitioner or Physician Assistant: The Ultimate Guide to Hiring, Educating, and Integrating an NP or a PA

Copyright 2017 by Roger T. Moore, MD

Published by Dermwise Incorporated
Elkhart, Indiana

ISBN 10:0-692-95105-9
ISBN 13: 978-0-692-95105-7

Legal Disclaimer

As a dermatologist my area of expertise is truly in the field of dermatology. That being said a legal disclaimer is necessary for the content of this book.

This book is not intended to be legal or ethical advice. It is a collection of opinions, mostly mine, experiences from my private dermatology practice, and input gained from other dermatologists, nurse practitioners, and physician assistants. Any information provided here should be reviewed by your lawyer, since duties and laws in regard to medicine, employment, and patient care vary from state to state. Any actions taken after reading this material are the sole responsibility of the one taking the action.

The author and publisher make no warranties, express or implied, about the materials or instruction provided within this book. The reader should review the legal and ethical rules within the jurisdiction he or she practices.

Contents

Part Four
Integration of an NP or a PA

Part Five
Where This Book Came from
and Where to Take This Knowledge

Introduction

If you have ever wondered where health care is going and asked yourself how you are going to keep up, then you are not alone. As the owner of a single specialty dermatology practice, I have found the changes and burdens of the new health care movement overwhelming, to say the least. Somehow I have been fortunate to be exposed to some savvy, successful businesspeople who have helped shed light on a course through these treacherous waters that we travel as physicians.

It is crazy, but living in the small town I have practiced in has afforded me the opportunity to meet and interact with many businesspeople who have grown their companies to incredible size and worth. The methods they have taught me have shown me an effective way that each dermatologist can grow their practice in his or her own town and medical community.

The culmination of many discussions about business growth, profitability, culture, and how to integrate and give back to a community have led me in guiding my own practice. At the same time, they have inspired me to write this book and guide, so that those who practice dermatology can have the hope to find similar or greater success.

The basic premise of providing excellent service and quality care are simply not enough anymore. Due, in part, to how the changes in health care laws are impacting them, patients are insisting upon more timely access to their doctors and better quality care. Plus, they have such high deductibles and other out-of-pocket expenses, they want, and even need, it done cheap. Unfortunately, cheap doesn't correspond to overhead expenses, which are escalating out of control. The doctor of today now has to find a way to become a businessperson, or else lose themselves to a life of paperwork and statistics, or give up and join the massive entities.

Whether you work for a multispecialty group, single specialty group, or are a solo dermatology practice, we are in this struggle together. The reasons we went into medicine are still the same, but the path to get there has changed. It is through the concerted effort we make together to improve our practices, the care we give, and the service we render, that we can make our jobs great again.

This book is a culmination of the transformation I made from being the doctor who denounced non-physician care, to a person who has found a way to train, educate, and integrate nurse practitioners and physician assistants, so that even some the most critical physicians can find acceptance of their utilization in dermatology practices.

The topic is one seen as a minefield, with no consensus from the powers that be in how to get the NP or PA to meet some standard. After devoting years to building an online training system, Dermwise, I designed this book to help lay the blueprint for those dermatologists who want to find stability in the crazy world of health care, or better yet—who want to grow their practices.

The benefits of having highly trained and qualified NP or PA on your team can be innumerable. I would even say there is some magic to be discovered in having a practice with an NP or a PA, if the process is approached right. We can always make adjustments, but we only get one shot at this life and this career. It is my sincere desire that this material will help you find joy and excitement to live the life you have desired. Together let's make this journey worth the ride.

May you be blessed with much peace, success, and happiness.

—Roger T. Moore, MD

Part One

Amid Modern-day Health Care Challenges,
the Proven Strategy of Success

Chapter 1
The Secret to Lasting Stability
of Practice and Income

Many dermatologists are not aware of an essential secret that secures long-term stability of a practice and its income. They think the farther out they are scheduled, the more secure their practice is. The fact is, the majority of dermatologists who read this book are leaders of dermatology in their communities. But without knowing this simple business truth, each is prime for competitors to plant themselves next door and bleed their business dry.

Only a small percentage of dermatologists figure out this unknown and use it to their advantage. Most do not see the unpleasant truth, which is evident to the giant health care organizations that employ so many primary care providers in their regions. Ignoring this truth leads to many patients obtaining a significant portion of their dermatology care at their primary care office or another setting. Some dermatologists consider this secret a ploy, and instead of using it, they resent it. They resist the fact a problem even exists.

That secret is this: The most stable and highest income earning practices *meet the needs of their patients.*

What do I mean by this? For decades the demand for dermatology services has steadily been on the rise. According to the American Cancer Society, the increasing occurrence of skin cancer is a primary driver of the rising demand for dermatology services. In addition, the population continues to grow older, including an entire generation of baby boomers now expanding the patient pool, and more of them are seeking dermatologic care.

There has long been a shortage of dermatologists, which is expected to persist for the foreseeable future. Because of this trend, accompanied by unrealistic healthcare regulatory burdens, many dermatologists are spread thin with these strict demands placed on their time and attention. Many find themselves overworked and overwhelmed. It is a common occurrence for dermatologists to have schedules booked out three or more months in advance. This makes it difficult for patients to get in to see their "skin doctor."

The number one tenet of meeting patients' needs requires being *accessible* to your patients. How you do this isn't the way a lot of providers might think. Most believe they can only see so many patients and do so much every day. The reality is, you can do more—and delegate more—than you thought possible.

Most patients would gladly be seen at their dermatologists' offices, even if they do not speak directly with the doctors every visit. Patients know and trust their dermatologists. They also respect the fact a dermatologist would not let someone represent his or her practice who is not competent. The majority of patients are happy to be under the care of a dermatology team member. They simply want access to quality care.

As the world of health care changes more and more, savvy dermatologists are exploring the possibility of hiring and training a nurse practitioner (NP) or a physician assistant (PA). A well-trained NP or PA can help get patients seen faster, treated more efficiently, and in so doing, better satisfy the needs of patients.

Plus, it can provide a vehicle for expansion of your services.

Many physicians use the nurse practitioners and/or physician assistants to see short-term follow-up patients, acute simple rashes, lesions (skin cancer screens), and routine chronic conditions such as acne, psoriasis, or rosacea. Some dermatologists need and utilize these providers as surgical assistants who can place sutures and help expand surgical services. Other dermatologists have them see only general dermatology patients, which increases the dermatologist's availability to perform surgeries or elective procedures.

NPs and PAs can care for dermatology patients, cosmetic patients, surgical patients, and more. This decreases the demand on a supervising physician's schedule to allow for more flexible hours, more free time, and allow for the physician to focus on the niche they prefer or manage more complex or demanding cases.

The addition of an NP or a PA provider may also allow the practice to extend clinical hours. All of these patient-centered benefits, including the addition of new services, if you desire, raise the level of patient care and therefore increase patient satisfaction . . . and positive patient reviews online as well as personal referrals. This will in turn generate more business.

What about cost? The fee schedules of NPs and PAs are often lower than those allowed for physicians. Since they generate revenues greater than their compensation expense to their employers, they are capable of generating revenue both for themselves and for the practice. Employing an NP or a PA who is properly trained is a sound business practice and is already being acknowledged by specialists as the way of the future in health care.

I truly believe this insightful discussion about hiring, training, and implementing an NP or a PA into a practice is sorely overdue. If this information had been laid out for me years ago, it could have saved hundreds of thousands of dollars, if not well in excess of seven figures.

In this book, you will be provided with the ultimate guide to hiring, training, and integrating an NP or a PA into your dermatology practice. This material has been gathered from a constellation of experiences from dermatologists who opted to work with nurse practitioners or physician assistants, and is coordinated to present proven steps to the successful implementation and utilization of NPs and PAs in the most efficient manner possible. This is a must-read for every physician who has contemplated hiring an NP or a PA, or who has identified the need to fortify his or her practice and take it to the next level. The information in this text removes the roadblocks that once held myself and others back.

I can assure you, if I knew all of what is known to me now during the early years of my practice, it would have bolstered the stability of my practice and made much more money. Though financial gain is not the end-all, it sure can put wind in the sails during long hours.

What I divulge to you through the coming pages is the findings of the work I poured my heart and soul into for fifteen-plus years. I am optimistic you will find know-how that will help you run a more efficient, stable, and profitable practice (and with less effort and a greater reduction in stress than you might imagine).

Chapter 2
What Is in a Title:
Nurse Practitioner

Before we delve into the crux of this book—how to efficiently and effectively hire, train, and integrate an NP or a PA into your practice—we will begin with a very brief overview of what a nurse practitioner and a physician assistant are. If you already know all the ins and outs of these providers, please feel free to skip this chapter and the next, but most physicians will discover new details worth knowing about, including their qualifications and backgrounds.

Nurse Practitioner (NP)

A nurse practitioner is an advanced practice nurse who has traditionally earned a master's or doctorate degree in nursing. Normally an NP has attained an undergraduate of nursing degree, where he or she is awarded a bachelor's degree in nursing and also obtains licensure to become a registered nurse. From here they often enter into a one- or two-year NP training program. The NP training program is typically a generalist degree in the realm of primary care, but may be focused on one specific area of medicine.

A variety of training specialties are recognized. Some of those more common areas include neonatal NPs, pediatric NPs, adult NPs, geriatric NPs, certified nurse midwives, women's health care NPs, family NPs, acute care NPs, certified registered nurse anesthetists, and others.

In some programs, individuals who have a bachelor's degree, but are not registered nurses, can combine training to obtain licensure as registered nurses and also sit for the certification boards as NPs at completion of the program. The rigors of this type of program often means they are highly selective in approving candidates.

NPs are trained to diagnose and treat a wide range of medical conditions. Dependent upon certain state laws, NPs are typically authorized to prescribe drugs in all fifty states, and they hold independent licenses to practice nursing either in collaboration with a physician or on their own.

The NP practice model, as reported by some experts, indicate a holistic approach to patient care with particular attention to risk reduction, disease prevention, and health promotion. This may be reflective of the National Organization of Nurse Practitioner Faculties (NONPF) core competencies guideline. The core competencies content described in 2017 for the NONPF website (www.nonpf.org) include the areas of scientific foundation, leadership, quality, practice inquiry, technology, information literacy, policy, health delivery system, ethics, and independent practice.

Though in the past most NPs obtained only masters' degrees, there is a trend among NP organizations that encourages NPs to work toward obtaining doctorate degrees. The doctor of nursing practice (DNP) is the current highest level of education for nurse practitioners. Some in the field of nurse practitioners mention they feel the DNP may become the standard.

What does all of this mean? The DNP, per a 2004 position statement from the American Association of College of Nursing (AACN), is both the terminal degree for clinical nursing education and the graduate degree for advanced nursing practice.

The DNP is focused on practice competencies rather than the PhD's in-depth focus on academic research.

The push for a higher degree by nurse practitioners tandems what some believe is a movement to gaining independent practices. Some NPs prefer independence, and a segment indicate a desire to become autonomous like physicians. Of note is that some states allow nurse practitioners to own their own practices. In this instance, a collaborative physician is often needed to review a small percentage of charts, but the practice is owned by the NP.

For more information, visit the American Academy of Nurse Practitioners website at www.aanp.org.

Chapter 3
What Is in a Title:
Physician Assistant

A physician assistant is a provider who has earned a master's degree through a physician assistant training program of general medical education. In most cases, a practicing PA is a nationally certified and state-licensed medical professional. A PA must also pass a national certifying exam administered by the National Commission on Certification of Physician Assistants. This certifies them, and the title is then Physician Assistant-Certified, or PA-C. Ongoing requirements must be met to maintain certification.

According to the American Academy of Physician Assistants (AAPA) website, the PA profession was created to improve and expand health care during the mid-1960s when a shortage of primary care physicians was noted. The first class of PAs was put together at Duke University Medical Center, where the initial class included former members of the military who had prior medical training. This first class graduated in 1967. Since that time PAs have become an accepted part of the medical community.

Many of the physician assistant programs require classes similar to those needed for admittance to medical school, such as chemistry, anatomy, biology, and microbiology. More than two thousand hours of clinical rotations are utilized, with an emphasis on primary care. This included family medicine, internal medicine, obstetrics and gynecology, pediatrics, general surgery, emergency medicine, and psychiatry. The rotations generally parallel medical school clinical rotations, which some physicians find a positive.

PAs have delegated prescriptive authority in all fifty states and can prescribe controlled drugs, depending on specific state laws.

A PA works in tandem with a supervising physician and complements the physician's ability to deliver a wide range of medical and surgical services to patients. Many physician assistants agree the role of their job is to act as a physician extender who will provide exemplary care in a strongly similar manner to the provider who employs them.

While PAs require supervision from a physician, they do not necessarily require the supervising physician to be physically present in the place where the services are being rendered, depending on state law. However, the physician and the PA must typically remain in contact, and the ability for a patient to be seen by the physician within a short period of time may be a state statute.

More information on PAs, including education, qualifications, and certification, is available at www.aapa.org.

Chapter 4
Is Hiring an NP or a PA
Right for Your Practice?

Certain questions will need to be answered to determine whether hiring an NP or a PA is right for your practice. These questions center around the patient needs and thus the practice needs, the space/office/staff capabilities, the time and energy you can put toward training, and more.

Am I booked one or two months out? In other words, is there a high enough demand for patient services that is not being met by the current physician and staff? A practice that has long wait times for patients to be seen is the first sign that hiring an NP or a PA provider may be a worthwhile venture.

Unfortunately, we dermatologists often get duped into thinking a long wait time is a good thing. In truth, the lengthy wait time narrows the patient demographics for a practice. The patients who can wait a few months will bring in conditions that are relatively stable, recurrent, or chronic in nature. However, the art of early diagnosis and utilization of dermatologic training to diagnose acute rashes, lesions, or syndromes is minimized.

Long wait times are not the ideal scenario for any patient and should not be for any medical practice. The two problems we find with long wait times are, one, the patients of a practice seek dermatologic care elsewhere, including their primary care office (which, in modern health care, often includes a nurse practitioner or physician assistant—who is not trained in dermatology). This disenfranchises patients and teaches them to contact a non-dermatology office for the initial evaluation. And two, as noted previously, long wait times make a practice susceptible to competition, as it is a great reason for another dermatology provider to come to the area, either by his or her own recognizance or via a hospital or health network wanting to satisfy its patient population.

If it takes a patient more than a month to get an appointment in your office, it is time to begin considering if hiring a nurse practitioner or physician assistant is best for your patients and thus practice. When starting the evaluation process, you should ask yourself the following questions.

Do I have the space? Can your practice spare extra exam rooms for another clinician? If your available rooms are limited, this may not be a deterrent. Consider altering days or times worked. For example, your NP or PA could work the mornings that you, the physician, do not normally work.

Am I prepared to absorb the overhead of additional salary until the NP or PA generates his or her own revenue? If the nurse practitioner or physician assistant is not already trained in dermatology, there is a learning curve. During this time, the new provider is not defraying overhead, but is part of overhead expenses. In addition, it can take months for insurance contractors to credential the provider, and longer yet for payments to come into the practice. The practice must absorb the salary of the new hire until revenue is generated.

You can learn more in Chapters 18 and 19.

Do I have time to train a provider? If the NP or PA does not have experience in dermatology, the astute physician will plan ways they will immediately enable the practice to function more smoothly while helping offset initial costs. After minimal training, this can include tasks like post-operative wound check/suture removals, calling back melanoma patients, writing letters to referring providers, functioning as a scribe for the physician while in the exam room, performing surgical assistant duties, and any other tasks that may be delegated and overseen. These reduce the supervising physician's workload so that the physician can be more efficient. The physician must determine what aspects of their day can flow more efficiently with another provider doing part of the work. The goal is efficiency and to free up the physician's schedule. This can also provide more time so he or she can train the NP or PA more quickly. All that said, the physician must first have time to do the initial training. Later in the book we will discuss tools and techniques to maximize efficiency of education, including the time-saving Dermwise online training system.

Is there a defined role and long-term plan for the nurse practitioner or physician assistant? It is beneficial for the practice to clearly define the role the NP or PA will play in the practice after their training is complete. At the same time, determine exactly what type of relationship you would like to have with the nurse practitioner or physician assistant, including how much involvement you will have in the care of their patients, once the NP or PA has completed training. Consider defining if they will be seeing patients at initial presentation (new or new problems) to the office or only managing patients with established diagnoses rendered by the physician. By clearly defining the role and expectations of the provider at the outset, you will be able to better understand who will suit your practice.

What are the laws in my state? It is key to understand state laws and practice guidelines. Take the time to look up your specific state's laws regarding nurse practitioner and physician assistants, since the laws are essential to determining supervision, prescribing, and delegation.

For more information on state laws governing scope of practice, see the following websites.

- For NPs: American Academy of Nurse Practitioners at www.aanp.org. There is typically a section on regulation including state-specific rules or guidelines.
- For PAs: American Academy of Physician Assistants at www.aapa.org. There is typically a section for resources to facilitate learning about state-specific regulations.
- State medical societies' websites should also have information on regulations and guidelines.

If you are wanting to hire an NP or a PA for a medical spa, it is also advisable to review state law on the procedures that can be performed, what type of supervision/collaboration is required, and what level of responsibility is mandated for each party. Some states require the "medical director" to be a physician and may limit delegation of procedures.

How do the current insurance carriers handle credentialing and reimbursement of an NP or a PA?

Knowing which insurance companies will allow credentialing of NPs and/or PAs in your area could affect your hiring decisions. Likewise, it is important to understand requirements for being able to bill independently (i.e., some insurances require physicians to have hospital privileges, so practices would want to evaluate for similar requirements for NPs and/or PAs).

Most major insurance providers will cover services rendered by an NP or a PA. Some insurers will reimburse directly for services rendered by the NP or PA (as they view the NP or PAs to be an independent provider), while others require that the NP or PA be directly linked to a physician. These are the two ways in which a practice can bill for services rendered by an NP or a PA. The related terms are as follows.

- "direct" billing—The insurance is billed directly for services provided under the NP or PA's own name and NPI number.

- "incident-to" billing—The claim is generated under the supervising physician's name and NPI number.

Normally, "direct" billing under the NP or PA's name and NPI number is reimbursed 85 percent of the physician fee schedule, and "incident-to" billing is reimbursed 100 percent of the physician fee schedule.

Medicare is the standard and reimburses at the rate of 85 percent of the physician-allowed amount, when the NP or PA services are rendered as "direct billing." Because some insurance companies vary from this, it is best to check with them to be clear on how they handle billing and coding for your NP or PA.

In addition, billing often ties in with the level of supervision and involvement of the physician. It is best to become very familiar with the definition of "incident-to" and ensure the practice is in complete compliance if utilizing this method.

In order to bill "incident-to" with Medicare, there are strict supervision and scope-of-practice requirements. It is equally important to check with each payer to determine the specific billing requirements for services provided by an NP or a PA.

More information on "incident-to" is shared in Chapter 17.

How do I plan to educate and ensure competence? Most physicians in the dermatology specialty have put in countless hours of study to be at the top of their classes in medical school and then continued this dedication during residency and in practice. It is difficult for them to think that someone who has less education and has not put in the same level of study is going to care for their patients.

Simply put, many dermatologists believe a patient should be seen by a physician. This is clearly the golden ideology most physicians come out of training believing. Although this is the ideal scenario, this belief does not always last. In many practices across the nation, the new dermatologist has a full schedule relatively quickly and soon finds patients are having to wait weeks, if not months, for an appointment. The limited time in a day does not allow the doctor to see all the patients who need dermatology services.

The dermatologist-/physician-only mentality leads to an issue of determining whether it is better practice to allow the patient to be seen by a primary care provider, expand the hours of work of the dermatologist, or train a nurse practitioner or physician assistant in dermatology.

It is a fact that many aspects of health care reform are pushing for the utilization of NP and PA providers, as previously indicated. This is a truth that physicians must realize. From here the physician must decide how to react to this changing dynamic. The growth of many practices will rely on the ability to adapt to the future of health care (rather than attempt to re-create the past).

Many nurse practitioners and physician assistants you might bring on board have a background of practicing primary care but never had a dermatology rotation. That can lead to the potential of inaccurate diagnosis and patients left with a treatment plan that is not accurate or fails. Getting a nurse practitioner or physician assistant competent enough that the dermatologist feels comfortable yielding care of their patients is a significant undertaking. It is one that requires a plan for education, shadowing, and mentoring.

The information and strategies you need to get an NP or a PA educated and integrated into your practice will be presented to you throughout the pages ahead. A well-trained provider will understand the principles of dermatologic diagnosis, management, and when to move the patient on to the dermatologist. He or she will treat patients in the manner the dermatologist would, and will carry your personal reputation.

Once a dermatologist understands that he or she can be the chief strategist who directs solving their patients' problems with the NP or PA they have trained, a barrier is overcome. The dermatologist can be responsible for and manage a team that provides solutions to the skin problems that come through their practice. Patients discover that the nurse practitioner or physician assistant has excellent knowledge and that they still have access to the dermatologist for questions. Patients are commonly appreciative of the rapid access to care, professional treatment, and team approach.

Chapter 5
Pre-plan to Yield Big Returns

Once you have reviewed the questions in the previous chapter and your answers to most suggest that it is time to consider hiring an NP or a PA, read on, as the remainder of the content is absolutely for you. If you are not sure whether the investment of time, energy, and resources involved in working with an NP or a PA is for you, then continue reading to understand how this model of health care delivery can be performed in a positive manner.

The question I am most often asked is, "When should I hire an NP or a PA?" In dermatology the answer is YESTERDAY. Why? Because you can serve your patient population better by offering faster, high-quality care with a well-trained NP or PA. When the hiring and training *process* is handled properly, the patients will be grateful you have provided them rapid access for their problems.

It is wise to understand the word "process." It takes a system—a step-by-step plan—to attract the best candidates, hire the optimal fit for your needs, and then ensure a solid foundation is laid for his or her success in your practice. Choosing to plan for this outcome is one of the most important decisions you will make. Here is a brief story to illustrate.

As a friend of mine and I drove along, he described to me building his new house. Barely keeping one hand on the steering wheel, he animatedly used any available fingers plus his free hand to air-draw the place. The magnificent two-story brown brick home, he said, stood on a field of grass behind a large porte-cochère (coach gate) at the main entrance so his guests would feel like dignitaries even during inclement weather.

Entering the home, one stepped onto a ballroom-sized white marble floor that shone all the way to the back wall where sunlight streamed through a two-story bank of windows. Beyond the windows, the awesome wonders of nature filled in with tall shade trees and flowering plants at their base. When you stepped close, you would see a meandering stream flow between them.

To the left an airy, open-concept kitchen showcased the most up-to-date appliances, immaculate cabinetry, granite countertops, and crown moulding. Adjacent to this was a dining room large enough to fit a royal family and their friends. Across the main room, a pair of open doors revealed a study lined floor to ceiling with fine wood bookshelves that had been custom made, piece by piece.

In the passenger seat, I envisioned every detail and anticipated the upcoming tour. As the car neared the home's driveway, my friend finished telling me the features of his home. He signaled his turn onto a concrete driveway, and I leaned forward to view all he had described.

We rolled up the driveway to the top of a hill. He put the car into park, and we stepped out.

I stared at hard, plain concrete with pipes sticking out, the foundation of his home. I nodded and produced a smile for my friend, but this was not the picture I had had in mind.

To bring about this dream home, he had built and completed the project, even before the foundation had been poured.

What does this have to do with adding an NP or a PA to your team? It is understanding a process. He had to build the home in his mind before starting actual construction. He needed to envision the end goal, with specific details, before it could exist in reality.

As medical providers, it is not uncommon to forgo some of the planning phase and act on gut feelings when adding lasers, services, or technology to our practices. Vendors often count on this behavior when utilizing high-pressure tactics to garner sales. After an expense has been incurred and a product delivered, the physician then "makes it work" in some form or fashion.

Most physicians are not trained, or give much effort, to become businesspeople. If they understand any business concept, it is simply that they make money each month. The overhead, copays, insurance denials, uncollected debt, and missed leads on phone calls (which is where prospective patients gain their initial firsthand impression of you and your practice) are not even considered. On top of these items, most doctors miss the boat on the fact that *relationships build businesses.*

And like it or not, the practices we run are businesses. In many businesses, the customer who comes in once and is thrilled will spend five to seven times more at the business over the course of their lifetime. That is huge! Plus, they will refer family and friends, whereas they will avoid and steer loved ones clear of businesses—and doctors—that dissatisfy them. The referrals of patients are earned, not given.

For us that means every provider should be focused on giving the absolute best care and providing an experience for the patient that meets their needs, solves their problems efficiently and promptly, and overall *exceeds their expectations.*

Does that mean our services have to be free or cheap? Absolutely not. Consider Disney. This is one of the grandest ventures in the world, which provides such a wonderful experience people often shell out much more money than they anticipated and do so gladly with smiles on their faces. There is no free lunch at Disney. But there is a lunch that will be remembered for a lifetime.

We might not be able to provide a Disney experience in our offices, but we can remember that the happy customer knows their provider is intelligent, works diligently for them, and places their interest and concerns at the pinnacle of each visit.

It is the person who leaves your establishment fully satisfied and willing to come back for their next problem who is the crux of the medical business.

We do enough to get our practices off the ground, fighting tooth and nail to make our businesses viable. If patients are not flocking to our offices, we work longer hours, make inroads with other providers (build referral networks), join service organizations, advertise, and take many other small yet cumbersome steps to make our businesses economically feasible. Often there is not a premeditated plan that can be systematically implemented to make it all happen, simply a desire to keep it going and an unwavering fight to not give up.

Somehow this works for many providers. A relentless nature and willingness to work 60 to 100 hours a week exists when we complete residency. Many providers overcome their missteps and mistakes by sheer hard work and the volume of hours.

Too many providers attempt the same approach when they hire NPs or PAs into their practices. Most never look at how they are going to utilize their NP or PA. They simply want to push the overflow to the new hire. The haphazard manner of the "just make it happen" philosophy soon becomes a source of frustration for both the new hire and the physician. Frequently an NP or a PA gets frustrated with the perceived disorganized methods, and simply feels empty at the job because the old philosophy of "just get it done" is being employed. The NP or PA is often a bright person who made a choice somewhere in their life that the 100-hour weeks required of physicians in training were more than they would sacrifice. Thus, when the provider asks them to act like a resident physician (who worked the 100-hour weeks), it does not take long for them to look for greener pastures.

(Note that many NPs and PAs who go in search of a dermatology practice are looking for a setting that allows them to have weekends off and a less demanding schedule.)

The truth of the matter is this: The quickest way to detract from your reputation and your practice is to hire the wrong NP or PA, and/or worse yet, hire the right one and turn them loose on your patients before they are ready.

If you don't think this is accurate, try it. Occasionally big entities like hospitals and large health networks miss the boat on training the nurse practitioners and physician assistants they hire into specialties. The result is they tarnish their reputations by placing providers in roles they are not ready for.

The lack of 1) a structured (and proven) hiring method, 2) a training system, 3) an implementation process, and 4) an ongoing marketing and patient-relation system damage many practices.

So, it is best to create a systematic approach that will provide you with the best potential candidates—the vital first step in this process—and then will ensure methodical training, comprehensive implementation, and effective patient-provider connection.

Even though the process of hiring, educating, and integrating a new hire can seem daunting, there are tools and techniques that can facilitate a smooth transition into your practice, as well as reduce frustration and save money. At the same time, a properly organized and constructed plan can yield a great deal of satisfaction, fulfill a practice need, and result in big returns on your investment long-term.

At this point, the challenge that even forward-thinking dermatologists face is understanding how best to hire, train, and implement a system that enables them to get an NP or a PA up and going in their offices. In the chapters that follow, you will be provided with effective hiring, training, integration, and marketing techniques developed and refined through years of my own experiences, those of my own NP and PAs, and knowledge gained by interviewing fellow dermatologists who have brought NPs or PAs into their practices.

Part Two

Hiring

Chapter 6
Draft a Profile of
Your Golden Candidate

The hiring of a provider into an office is likely the most important hire a practice will ever make. The ideal NP or PA can be a rejuvenating addition to an office, and can ignite fresh energy, growth, and monetary rewards. Hiring the right person takes more than wishful thinking. It requires premeditated planning and holding to carefully thought-out criteria.

In dermatology, the number of applicants who state they have a "strong desire to practice dermatology" is typically very high. At the same time, the number of applicants who back up that assertion with action steps (like attending dermatology conferences, mentioning dermatology journals or books they have read, volunteering time shadowing a dermatologist, or other signs of commitment) are few and far between.

Most applicants do not have dermatology experience other than possibly one rotation in training. The "process" then becomes a means to sort through those who think working 8 to 5 is all that dermatology is about, to find the NP or PA who is truly dedicated to the specialty (though, as I recently pointed out, expecting them to work 100 hours per week should not be your goal either). The right candidate has strong intellectual capacity with enough conviction and wherewithal to commit to learn and practice dermatology.

The ideal candidate would come in already trained in dermatology and have worked in an office that deemed education as a cornerstone of the practice. In this setting, you might be able to hire and allow them to see patients rather quickly. Even in these instances, you should spend time overseeing, discussing plans, sharing patient visits, and reviewing charts at a higher rate than required by state law. You want to make sure that the two of your practice styles mesh well and that the same high level of care you provide is present.

The real-world occurrence, however, is often that candidates do not have the experience you would desire and you have to find the right personality, work ethic, and academic ambition to take on the demands of learning a specialty and then practice exactly like you want.

Knowing the type of person you would expect to thrive in the NP/PA role for your practice—and its culture—is key to helping you envision, and eventually hire, the right person.

Begin by considering your unique office culture. Office culture is your team's collective thought processes, values, and attitudes, as initiated and exemplified by you, the physician, and which your patients observe and experience. Next, describe for yourself the type of patients you expect the provider to see. You may find it helpful to write or keyboard this information, as well as your answers to the following, in a document so that you can use it to help you create a profile for your ideal provider.

You, as a physician, should always *be the person* you would want *to be seen by*. This philosophy should be sought out in new hires as well.

Define the Role of Your Future Provider

The best way to find the optimal NP or PA for your specific practice is to first decide what the role of that future provider will be. This step requires some forethought. It is important to envision what your practice will look like several months after the hire, including what the work relationship/expectations will be and how that provider will fit the specific culture of your practice.

It is helpful to ask yourself questions so that you can decipher this future view of your practice and the provider's role in it.

- What type of patients will they be expected to see?
  - New patients?
  - New diagnoses?
  - Cosmetic cases?
  - Surgical cases?
- Immediately after being hired, will the NP or PA see patients independently or alongside the physician?
- If the NP or PA will initially see patients alongside the physician, how long before the physician would like the provider to be seeing patients independently?
  - If seeing new diagnoses or new patients, what will determine their ability to see patients on their own?
  - When, if they are going to see cosmetic or surgical patients, can they see them independently?
- What is their list of duties?

Add to this list any other factors that help you clearly define the role of your future provider in your dermatology practice.

Define the Background and Qualifications of Your Future Provider

Questions you might consider about the experience of the future provider include the following.

- Does an NP or a PA fit our practice better?
- What type of medical background will best prepare him or her for our office?

- New graduate, one who has completed rotations or worked in another field (i.e., ER, family practice, or some other field showing they have basic clinical experience).
- Proficient provider with dermatology experience only.
- Could clinical practice in the nursing realm be ideal?
- Is it important for him or her to have research experience?
- Would prior work in a non-medical field be helpful?

Questions that define the NP or PA's predisposition to learning should be considered. Following are some sample questions to ask yourself.

- Are there didactic lessons they must complete?
- Will they read journals and periodicals on their own (outside of clinic)?
- Will he or she be someone who will present didactic material to the physician and/or other staff?
- How independent do they desire to be, and are they willing to self-educate as much as needed in order to achieve that outcome?

Add to this list any other factors that help you clearly define the background and qualifications of your future provider so that he or she will be the optimal fit for your dermatology practice.

Define the Character of Your Future Provider

What personality traits are important and do you expect your future hire to have?

Finding the right NP or PA requires matching the provider with not only the right experience to fit a role but also success tendencies that indicate he or she has what it takes to do well. Consider drafting a spec sheet on your optimal candidate, one that includes desired personality traits to fit your office culture as well as the following.

- ✓ possesses a strong drive
- ✓ displays a pattern of leadership
- ✓ has unwavering medical curiosity

Drive

When someone has a strong drive to perform well in their chosen field, it is displayed in their past and current situations as an unconditional commitment to excellence. Characteristics of someone with drive include the following.

- A history of success. The ideal person will often be goal-oriented, motivated, and have a tendency to get the job done.
- Unconditional commitment to goal attainment and/or professional advancement. This person can share with you several challenges they have overcome to get to their current position.
- Resilience. Patients unaccustomed to NPs and PAs are not always accepting of the new provider and/or their recommendations. A candidate with long-established resilience is one who maintains their confidence in the face of opposition and demonstrates willingness to overcome challenges.

Leadership

The right candidate should naturally guide and direct patients and staff, plus they do so in a way that reflects your own positive approach. They should also exhibit independence in many of their actions, as you do.

Additional traits for success in this area can vary, but essential characteristics include the following.

- Takes responsibility. Accepting challenges and responsibility is essential. A medical provider must take ownership for their decisions. This should be accompanied by a mind-set that finds answers to problems. They do not hunt for excuses but rather solutions to overcome challenges.
- Awareness. A great fit is someone who can maximize their own potential while also understanding their shortcomings. They may reveal this while sharing with you how they have overcome challenges (which additionally shows resourcefulness). Awareness as a leader also means they have helped others find success.
- Unwavering optimism. The person who can excel in a practice must be aware that their attitude is infectious to others. The ability to handle challenges in a positive way can contribute to the entire office response and outlook. (For example, how would the NP or PA handle being overbooked by the front office staff and running behind?)
- Trustworthiness is a must. The ability to be relied on as a truthful and honest person largely defines a true leader. Though every person might consider him- or herself trustworthy, traits that exemplify this can be identified. They include the ability to listen carefully to others, confidence paired with humility (they have experience but also the wisdom to ask for feedback), calmness, loyalty, and responsibility.

Medical Curiosity

The optimal NP or PA will possess an unwavering medical curiosity and a drive to learn. Each medical provider who is successful must take time outside of work to read, expand knowledge, and find answers to questions, and do so on an ongoing basis. Independence is a prerequisite for medical curiosity. You can identify medical curiosity in multiple ways, including the following.

- Knowledge finder. It is imperative that an NP or a PA can show they are willing to look up answers for complicated diagnostic entities. This ties in with the qualities of independence and responsibility. Without the attribute of knowledge finding, the candidate will not provide excellent care to your patients.
- Read on their own. A stellar NP or PA will read without being asked to read. This is a telltale sign the candidate takes the care of their patients seriously. There should be an answer when you ask what journal or medical book they have read most recently and when.

The above items can help identify the traits of a high performing NP or PA. At the same time, the person should have a set of skills plus experience enough to help the practice as quickly as possible.

Consider making your own list of "must-haves" for your future provider. These are traits that you desire in your perfect NP or PA. The following list is a brief example of what might be considered in the realm of skills, aptitudes, and experience.

Skills

- Strong grasp of the field of medicine as well as technology and trends.
- Exceptional presentation and communication skills that will enable them to provide clear and concise medical care.
- Excellent interpersonal skills displayed by their ability to establish rapport, build relationships, and participate in activities.

Aptitudes

- Intelligence. This can be noted in transcripts of undergraduate and graduate degrees. What the candidate said, did not say in their communication with you, and how they communicate, may also display this.
- An enduring can-do attitude.
- Self-starter. It is important to find candidates who display the ability to be self-motivated and self-directed.

Experience

- Minimum of a completed NP or PA training program.
- __ years' experience in ER, urgent care, primary care, or another field.
- __ years' experience in dermatology (optional).
- In lieu of above-mentioned experience, has taken courses in dermatology.
- Has completed training in dermatology, such as a dermatology conference, volunteered in a dermatology office, or completed online dermatology training (i.e., Dermwise Quick Start Online Dermatology Training, a program developed by the author of this book and utilized by many dermatologists).

The lists in this chapter can be used as guides to making sure you find the optimal NP or PA candidates. Interview questions, which will be discussed in detail in an upcoming chapter, can be tailored around the items you feel are most important.

When you create a detailed vision of what you want the end result to be, you will be able to attract the strongest candidates. Thus, it is important to take the time to give this deliberate thought before writing the job ad, which will also be detailed in an upcoming chapter. Once you have a clear vision of who the ideal candidate will be to help expand and grow your practice, the process of writing the ad, sorting through the resumes, and conducting interviews can be completed much more smoothly.

The goal is to find the absolute best fit for your organization so they will be excited to be part of your team, feel that they belong, and will achieve success for him- or herself as well as your practice. When you plan ahead by creating a list of golden criteria for your future hire, you are much more likely to hire the right person, the first time.

Chapter 7
Evade These Pitfalls
to Ensure a Great Hire

Hiring an NP or a PA can be unlike anything else we do on a daily, monthly, or annual basis. The investment in money, time, and effort required to get the new hire up to speed and integrated into the practice (even if they have experience) can be enormous for the entire office staff. It is clearly an area where errors in judgement with regard to getting the right person can be devastating to all involved.

In running a solo practice, I have had the opportunity to be involved in almost every aspect of the practice. Hiring has been one of those areas. Since it is so important, I have continued to remain involved in hiring, even after fifteen years of work. Why do so when my days are already busy? Because the process of hiring is crucial to the success of our practice.

Mistakes in this realm are so costly that they can deteriorate the morale of the entire team who is working with you. I have watched our staff get frustrated when a new medical assistant spends months being trained without catching on or takes excessive time off work. The spirit of the office can drop, and the practice runs the risk of having excellent team members getting dissatisfied and leaving. In addition, a poor hire can underwhelm your patients. And believe me, patients can tell when you do or do not have an outstanding NP or PA.

Now when we think of hiring an NP or a PA, it is not only the medical assistant/nursing staff who can get frustrated with incompetency. It is the administrative team, scheduling issues, and most importantly, *you*, the supervising physician, that can suffer consequences day after day. That is right—we as physicians are the ones training, educating, and investing our time to get them up to speed. So avoiding missteps in this realm is key.

Common missteps in the hiring process can be found in the following.

- Being fooled by a great resume. Rather than correctly gauge the resume as the first of many tools, many professionals who hire weigh the resume too heavily in the decision-making process, as if it is the primary tool. Be aware: The resume is often helpful and can give insight into the past, but it almost never reflects how the person will perform in your office.

- Going with the gut feel. Though intuition can be beneficial in certain circumstances, when hiring a provider there are necessary steps and requirements that must be in place to ensure fit and competency. The gut feel must be placed in proper perspective.

- Hiring because a friend referred. The judgement of friends and colleagues is not the problem, but rather our assumption that their recommendation makes a provider an accurate fit for the specific role, background, traits, and culture fit that we need in our practice.

- Overvaluing experience in the specialty. Hiring a competitor's NP or PA might be the best thing you could do . . . for your competitor. Experience is not always as valuable as one might think, particularly if the person has not been trained well. More valuable than specialty experience is avoiding poor training or bad practices being placed into your business.

- Believing their stated desire. After years of hiring and growing a practice, I have encountered one common, recurrent thread: the number of NP or PAs who state how deeply they want to do dermatology. Ninety-nine percent of the time, these same people do not own a dermatology text, willingly obtain any education in the field, or know more about the specialty than when they graduated. It is advisable to value deeds, not words, in this regard.
- Going on the "likeability" factor. Some people have such pleasing personalities that we may bypass red flags or avoid being as objective as we should be. Be sure to intentionally differentiate between likeability and performance.
- Using the standard questions for interviews. If you have interviewed people before, you know that questions about strengths and weaknesses often yield similar responses among prepared candidates. Such responses tell you whether a person has prepared for the interview, though not much more. Develop interview questions that focus on aspects of the candidate that compel them to be, well, candid about who they really are and what they truly want in their careers. More on specific topics and items to ask are discussed in the interviewing section of this book.

A practice can hire genuinely nice and good-natured people while using the steps above as the backbone of their decision-making process.

The unfortunate truth is that bad hiring practices are all too common. It is in your best interest to treat the sequence of this addition/hire with the level of respect, detail, and planning it deserves. In the following chapters, we will discuss how to avoid the above missteps and what to do to take control of the hiring process. You will be given tools to facilitate a professional, organized, and efficient hiring process.

Chapter 8
Did You Know the Term
"Mid-Level" Provider Is Offensive?

Before you place an ad and start communicating with potential candidates for your position, it is best to learn a bit about terminology.

There are obvious distinctions between nurse practitioners and physician assistants. They are trained differently, are accustomed to different organizational structures, and they have varied political influences.

At the same time, many physicians "lump" the two together because their functionality is similar within the medical office setting. Unbeknownst to some physicians, there is a political correctness that comes when referring to NPs and PAs together.

Most physicians have utilized the term "mid-level" provider when referring to a nurse practitioner or physician assistant. The term has long been used to render a distinction between a physician, who has a medical degree and often completed a residency, from the NP or PA, who does not attain a four-year medical degree (MD) or typically complete residency training in their specialty. To most physicians, the term has been used without any negative connotation intended.

However, there is a strong movement in the health care industry, led primarily by the nurse practitioners, to remove the term "mid-level" provider and replace it with something more along the lines of "advanced practicing provider (APP)" or "physician extender (PE)."

The concern from health care providers is that the term "mid-level" can be interpreted as suggesting that only partial care or middle-level care is being administered by the "mid-level" provider. The fact that a patient's trust might be reduced when their provider is referred to as "mid-level" has been of concern. Some professionals have suggested the term be abolished.

Many nurse practitioners and the leadership of the American Academy of Nurse Practitioners (AANP) have strong opinions on this topic, which I have learned from personal experience. While I served as an exhibitor at a regional AANP meeting in Chicago for our business, the course director took exception to the term "mid-level" in our brochure and booth signage . . . so much so that she asked us to remove all items with the term on it. I learned quickly that this term does not merely bother some NP or PA providers, but that they take extreme exception to it.

I bring up this topic to make sure you are aware of the tension this term may cause in some circles. The title "advanced practicing provider," "physician extender," or simply "nurse practitioner" or "physician assistant" is typically seen as more acceptable and conveys the level of care that patients need to associate with your practice in order to continue to hold it in high regard.

Chapter 9
Create a Detailed Job Description

The Power of a Job Description

When setting out to hire the NP or PA who will best fit your practice, create a detailed job description that clearly states what you want your NP or PA to do. This explicit job description will be invaluable throughout the hiring process. Since it also provides the new hire a guide for their responsibilities, it leaves no room for guesswork and ensures the NP or PA will be accountable during employment. To extend that point, a great job description can be used in the future for performance appraisals and compensation reviews.

Therefore, be sure to put time into building a solid job description for your NP or PA. A highly effective job description specifies the following.

Job Title:
Reports to:
General Job Description:
Performance Criteria:
Education and Other Requirements:

We will look at these points one at a time. The following are ideas and considerations for details to include. Tailor them to your own specifications.

Job Title: Advanced Practice Nurse (or Physician Assistant)

Reports to: Medical Director/Collaborating Physician/Supervising Physician*

*NPs often refer to it as collaborating. PAs often refer to it as supervising. Your state medical society may factor into this.

General Job Description:

   The nurse practitioner (or physician assistant) functions to expand the provider role in coordination with supervising (or collaborating) physician. The NP (or PA) takes history, evaluates, performs dermatologic examinations, creates assessments, and formulates plans for patients of the practice. The NP (or PA) orders appropriate tests and biopsies as indicated medically. Care administered will be as appropriate for the standards of the practice and nationally. May have responsibility for education, research, and administrative services.

Performance Criteria:

PRIMARY JOB RESPONSIBILITIES

   a. Utilize dermatologic assessment skills and knowledge of clinical therapeutics to evaluate, diagnose, and manage/treat patients of the practice.

   b. Educate patients regarding dermatologic conditions, therapies, risk factors, and preventative care.

   c. Be knowledgeable in and able to perform ordering of appropriate diagnostic tests and therapeutic interventions.

   d. Prescribe appropriate pharmacologic therapeutic agents while stratifying risks and educating patients regarding risks.

   e. Assist in surgical and elective procedures as well as manage wound-care patients according to practice standards.

   f. Demonstrate competency in the management of emergency situations in a professional and calm manner.

   g. Maintain continuity of patient care through follow-up, monitoring response to therapies, and modifying plans as medically indicated.

   h. Coordinate communication with referring providers.

   i. Identify needed resources for the practice and care of patients.

   j. Supervise and manage the support staff (i.e., medical assistants) and others as assigned while reporting to office manager.

k.   Perform other duties as assigned or required.*

*It is always best to include in the job description a line indicating the NP or PA will need to handle "duties as assigned." Candidates must understand that the job description provided is neither all-inclusive nor immutable.

RESPONSIBILITIES TO ENSURE PATIENT SATISFACTION
a.   Promote a positive, patient-oriented work environment.
b.   Exhibit positive verbal and nonverbal communication skills.
c.   Acknowledge and respond to patient requests and calls promptly and courteously.
d.   Maintain and ensure other staff are maintaining confidentiality of patient, employees, and hospital information following HIPAA guidelines.

TEAMWORK AND LEADERSHIP
a.   Be a team player who sets an example for others in working together.
b.   Motivate and actively work with others in the role of mentor and supervisor, including oversight of delegated responsibilities.
c.   Serve as OSHA and HIPAA officer for the practice.
d.   Supervise within appropriate safe practice standards.
e.   Demonstrate respect, appreciation, and sensitivity for the patients and staff.
f.   Organize, prioritize, schedule, and manage work and responsibilities of self and staff to maximize productivity and be timely in duties while maintaining high-quality care.

g. Learn all steps involved in any task that is delegated.

h. Routinely perform tasks correctly the first time, with minimal waste of time and resources, and ensure staff are doing the same.

i. Take accountability for own actions and results.

FLEXIBILITY, ADAPTABILITY, AND INFORMATION MANAGEMENT/COMMUNICATION

a. Demonstrate an openness to change and flexibility to support the practice in its endeavors to provide exceptional care.

b. Accept constructive feedback and act upon suggestions provided to improve.

c. Effectively communicate and document issues of staff and patients.

d. Report conditions of patients to supervising physician and referring provider in appropriate manner for information they should know.

e. Use computer documentation, communication, and application efficiently, and ensure staff does so as well.

f. Keep manager updated and informed of daily operation and policy issues.

The above statements reflect the core duties of this job and responsibilities. Note that they are not a complete description of all work requirements inherent to the position.

As noted above, depending on the size of your office, you might give thought to requiring your NP or PA to be a liaison or officer for HIPAA or OSHA. As a liaison your provider would help the office maintain compliance with state and federal laws to protect office stability. In working with HIPAA, the provider can contribute input regarding rules on who a practice can fax information to, when records can be faxed, and what documentation is required. Who should be the most knowledgeable person for this? The provider, whether it is the physician, NP, or PA. Providers should understand medical requests the best.

So, consider having your NP or PA play a role in this process of HIPAA. Why? One, they are salaried and can answer questions before and after their shift, if needed. Two, it is a role that relates directly to patient care. Three, they are usually very responsible individuals who can help the practice maintain compliance. Four, they are typically present when patient care activities occur and thus likely to be available when questions arise.

Another office role would be to oversee a component of OSHA. The providers might be able to ensure medical personnel wear closed-toe shoes, do not have food in inappropriate locations, and other occupational safety requirements.

Though many of these duties will require the physician's or officer manager's supervision, having providers involved in compliance can add a layer of stability.

Education and Other Requirements:

MINIMAL EDUCATION:	Masters of Nursing (or Physician Assistant)
REQUIRED CERTIFICATION:	Certified as Nurse Practitioner (or Physician Assistant)
REQUIRED LICENSES:	Licensed as Advanced Practice Nurse or Physician Assistant. Must have qualification, or be able to qualify, for (state) and DEA prescribing numbers.

A solid job description for your practice may include all of the above items, or more items, or fewer. Of utmost importance is to outline the details of what is expected before the hire.

Some other items to consider including in the job description would be the following.

- Details regarding the NP or PA's scope of work, such as giving injections, suturing wounds, overseeing photodynamic therapy, supervising UVB therapy, participating in or supervising cosmetic/elective procedures, or other healing measures your practice performs and your NP or PA will need to undertake.
- A requirement for continuing medical education (CME), maintenance of licensure, hospital/medical society requirements, and CPR certification.
- Specifications for equipment the NP or PA must operate (i.e., surgical apparatus, laser, UVB, computers, etc.).
- Physical requirements.

- Sites of practice the applicant must travel to, such as hospitals or satellite offices.

Note: You may find job descriptions and templates through a variety of online resources. The Medical Group Management Association (MGMA—www.mgma.com) is a resource used by our office and was reviewed for some of the content in this chapter.

Chapter 10
Write a Job Advertisement to *Repel* (and to Attract)

Your advertisement needs to repel. Repel? Yes, that is right. It should repel the wrong candidates and attract the right candidates. If you are like me, the NP or PA who thinks they are doing me a favor by staying after 5:00 p.m. to finish charting or to answer messages is better off working for someone else. This is not to say there are days we would all like to be out of the office efficiently, but the reality is the hourly mentality is not what makes a successful health care provider.

Why is this mentioned here? Well, a great number of practices hire nurse practitioners. Reaching this position typically starts with a person working many years as an hourly employee. The mentality of working a set number of hours can be ingrained in some of these candidates. A leap in responsibility and a shift in thinking is essential for those who do not already possess this approach when they become a provider.

Most practices need providers who are concerned about patient care before the time clock.

In 1937, Napoleon Hill wrote the book *Think and Grow Rich*. While conducting research for his book, he met and interviewed some of the most successful and influential people of his era, including steel magnate Andrew Carnegie, inventor Thomas Edison, and automobile tycoon Henry Ford. During this process, Hill identified a series of success principles. One that he described is how successful people go beyond the call of duty and provide more service than what is called for or paid for. He wrote that the habit of doing this is crucial to success.

In my opinion, as influenced by Hill, any professional who is going to master a craft must first put in hours beyond the work week to gain knowledge to be proficient. For this reason, in our advertisements we make it clear that a great deal of study is expected. During the interview process, this point is underscored and discussed. When we hire someone with no dermatology experience, there are no misunderstandings in terms of the expected commitment to master the specialty of dermatology. Thus, with my strong convictions, I make it clear a provider should put in time outside of clinic hours to read and educate themselves. You would gain long-term from taking a similar approach.

A predisposition to learning is key. Though the optimal candidate may not always be available when you need them, the right person can be converted into the right candidate. The right person must be willing to not only take direction, but also undergo your training and demonstrate a mind-set of *continual* learning.

In addition, the right candidate will possess a high level of self-sufficiency.

Therefore, the advertisement must be designed to repel the person who is wanting the easy hours of dermatology clinic without the grueling hours of study.

Once that is tactfully made clear, be sure to attract the right candidates. Offer them an opportunity to learn, be mentored, and master a specialty. From a business perspective, it is up to the supervising physician to meet and exceed patient expectations, and to intentionally hire for and exemplify that stance. Oftentimes the right personality and disposition is the key to success within the practice setting. Finding a person who has values similar to yours and those of the practice makes for a better fit, which is more manageable than someone with differing values. So, reveal through your writing the personality (unique culture) of your office environment, the level of patient care you provide, as well as highlights of working with you personally (such as patient and thorough teacher, or positive, upbeat personality).

Attract the optimal candidate. The person who reads the job posting and feels like you are describing them and their ideal job is likely the person who fits your practice.

In this day of electronic media, many avenues of advertisement, including most avenues mentioned in the following section, do not charge per word for the advertisement. For this reason we can describe what is expected, what type of candidate we want, and any other components for the job, in as much detail as necessary.

A sample of a job posting follows. We have used a similar ad. (Note: Our ad was placed under the heading of "dermatology nurse practitioner or physician assistant" at www.indeed.com.)

Tremendous Opportunity for a Nurse Practitioner or Physician Assistant!

Dermatology office in (city, state) is hiring a special Nurse Practitioner or Physician Assistant.

Experience life the way it was meant to be. A working environment where you can look forward to the people you work with, the type of work you do, and the patients you care for. You have a choice to be the best, and you deserve the best in your career.

The supervising physician is friendly and treats his patients like family. The hand-picked staff are equally

---

welcoming, and the newly renovated office is a bright, uplifting environment.

Working in dermatology provides daily satisfaction, as our patients are pleasant, have an appreciation for outstanding care, and appreciate being seen in a timely manner, which you help provide. This specialty is one with a quality lifestyle, since there are rarely weekend office hours and call. If you do not have experience in dermatology, you will be trained.

Your specific duties will include:

- Together with the supervising physician, provide coordinated and shared care for general dermatology patients.
- Manage your immediate support team.

Upon completion of training (to be determined by hiring physician), your additional duties will include:

- Care for your own patients, from initial presentation to completion of visit.
- Assist in surgery and post-operative follow-ups.
- Contribute to OSHA safety requirements and/or oversee compliance in the office.
- Duties as assigned.

You will need to read a considerable amount, since you must obtain a strong knowledge base to be a quality dermatology provider long-term. You will receive some time during your work schedule to read the first few months. However, you will also be expected to read outside of clinic time. The demands of work are heavy intellectually, and you must be committed to a future in dermatology or you are not the right fit.

If you are a dedicated, hard-working individual who is passionate about becoming the best at what you do, you should consider this opportunity. There is a need for dermatology services here, so job security is high. Great local and regional activities await you and those important to you.

Dr. Moore is the founder of Dermwise training, an online dermatology training system utilized by hospitals and dermatology practices nationwide. Participating in this innovative educational process is included when you join our team. Learn about this training at www.dermwise.com.

If you feel this is the right job for you, send a cover letter with your contact information and resume via mail to (address) or e-mail to (e-mail address). If by e-mail, place your name in the subject line, along with the words *NP* (or *PA*) *Opening*. In your cover letter, please describe why you would be willing to live in this location, why dermatology is your field of choice, and what work you have done in dermatology already. If you e-mail us, make sure you get a follow-up e-mail confirming receipt. All inquiries are confidential.

Note that the advertisement contained specific instructions in terms of how to apply. It states that if an e-mail is rendered, then a particular subject line is to be typed in. It requires that the applicant provide a cover letter, whether responding by e-mail or snail mail. Details like these are tools. They provide a method to determine who is going to follow instructions and put forth effort, and who is not.

The quality of an applicant's cover letter and resume will also provide you with great clues into their ability to expertly articulate their thoughts, which they will need to do as a provider.

While I wrote this book, one candidate who responded to the posting for our office had a decent resume but wrote a two-page cover letter that rambled and bordered on incoherent at times. Another resume was sent in with no cover letter and simply the line "I have seen Dr. Moore at the hospital and would like to apply for his position." I received these letters the same week as another candidate's, who wrote a very succinct, articulate, and professional cover letter. It was obvious from the cover letter alone which candidate put time and thought into the application.

You can determine how much value you place on the cover letter, resume, and the attention to detail. You are hiring someone to be an extension of your image and practice. The ability to follow directions, communicate clearly, and present ideas in a favorable manner are important considerations that begin revealing themselves in these first items of correspondence.

Include these pointers in your job advertisements so that you may bypass the wannabes and pinpoint the high-end candidates.

This is a key step in the systematic approach to identifying the right type of candidate and maximizing the efficiency with which you perform your search. Remember, you are working to repel the candidates who would not be a good fit and attract the ones who will enhance the quality of your practice.

Following are the top four items I have found particularly advantageous to include in the job description.

1. List directives. Those who follow directions are the providers I prefer. This method helps identify this trait.
2. Require a cover letter. Besides learning who follows directions, the information obtained in the cover letters can help the strong candidates distinguish themselves.
3. Emphasize there will be expected reading outside of clinic. This sets the tone for the expectations I will have

for a provider. It repels those who have a nine-to-five mentality, while it resonates with those who are committed to a new specialty and understand the educational endeavor required.

4. Share that the quality of training has been extremely beneficial. We always reveal that candidates will be trained with the Dermwise training system (www.dermwise.com). This has consistently attracted high-quality and intellectual candidates. The candidates we feel are a superior fit for our practice are magnetically attracted to the concept of a strong educational program.

As you can see, the value of the advertisement is not in obtaining responses. It is in obtaining the right candidates who respond the proper way. The details presented in this type of advertisement can neatly exclude all would-be candidates except the detail-oriented, driven, and intellectual providers who communicate well.

Although I stressed this point previously, I want to accentuate it once more: Invest the time to write a strong job ad. Your training of the new hire during the first months or year will be infinitely easier when you utilize well-planned techniques during the hiring process. A little time spent now can pay huge dividends in the future.

Chapter 11
Get the Word Out
to Get the Resumes In

When your job description is complete and you are ready to begin the search for your candidate, you need to get word out that you are hiring. Several modalities are available. The region you reside in may dictate the terms of effectiveness.

- Place an advertisement in a local newspaper(s). The cost can be high, and reaching the professionals in the area may not be optimal, depending on the circulation and readership.
- Place an advertisement in a local newspaper(s) online. I have experienced success with this option by attracting local candidates when others did not want to relocate to my region of the country.
- Use a general online job site. Many dermatology practices, including our own, have had favorable results with these. There are multiple job sites available, which can be found with a quick Internet search. At the time of writing this book, the site Indeed.com is one of our most used modalities. Sites such as Monster.com, Careerbuilder.com and others are good options.
- List your job opening at Health eCareers (www.healthecareers.com). At the time of this writing, the American Academy of Dermatology utilizes the AAD Career Compass online job posting site through Health eCareers. You must pay to advertise in this venue, but the applicants do not have to pay, so it can be helpful.

- Post free advertisements through regional, state, and/or national societies. The Society of Dermatology Physician Assistants provided our practice a free advertisement in their online job postings. Our state dermatologic society also placed a free ad for our position on their website. Neither of these restricted word count.
- Contacting regional NP or PA training programs to find out the sites they recommend can also be helpful at identifying local or current trends.
- Local NPs or PAs can provide insight on where they look for jobs.
- Contact nurse-practitioner- or physician-assistant-certification programs in the area. If you know in advance you are going to hire, you can ask for a list of people interested in dermatology and offer to rotate several for a period of time. Having a rotator helps you get to know the candidate, including their intellect, personality, and interaction with patients and staff. This model requires more time up front but can pay off nicely if the right hire is made.

Send them a letter that includes your detailed job description and the location. These programs may simply post your advertisement for a short time, so you may prefer to send the letter every month until you fill the position.

Even better is when you can find a program director or administrative staff member who knows the students. Do not be afraid to explain the type of student you are looking for. The staff member may be able to provide you with candidates who closely match your requirements. Most of this can be done through e-mails, so it is not too time consuming.

- Go through a medical recruiter. This can be particularly helpful if your goal is to locate an NP or a PA with experience. Fees range considerably, and the cost can be significant, as high as $20,000 for a placement in your practice, so it is best to discuss all fees and schedules before utilizing the service of a recruiter.

Some recruitment agencies will require a fee before a hire is made and then possibly more money when you do hire a provider, but if they find someone, it might be worth the price. Other agencies only charge if you hire the provider they sent you.

If you opt to make this type of investment, consider having a lawyer review the agreement and stipulating partial repayment if the hire does not last a specified time.

To extend that point, make sure there is a clause that addresses the issue of a new hire leaving the practice. If, for any reason, the new hire does not stay longer than a certain period (for example, as little as a few months, or as much as a year), a resolution should be outlined in the agreement that ensures fair treatment and compensation for all parties.

Note that in some regions of the country, getting quality, experienced NPs or PAs via a medical recruiter may be difficult. Part of this may be due to the fact that an agency may or may not spend much to market your position. Thus, it is worthwhile to read reviews of each prospective agency online before contacting them so that you omit all but the most effective recruiters.

Also remember even the most successful companies and hiring agents do not always make the right hire. On top of this, life changes as do people, so no hire is guaranteed to be permanent.

- Contact a pharmaceutical representative. After thinking about paying for a recruiter and the large amount of money they might want, you might be happy to know about the pipeline of free resources in the pharmaceutical representative world. Part of a drug rep's job is to help you succeed, and what better way than to fill your open position? The contacts drug reps have can be impressive, and they may very well be willing to do some legwork to at least bring you leads, who from their pool of contacts is likely to be someone with experience.

- Ask your current NP or PA, if you have one, to recommend a colleague of their acquaintance. If they are happy, they might gladly share a friend's name whom they feel would be good to work with. In addition, they may be willing to use their contacts, such as their school administrators, to help get the word out in a more well-received manner than you might secure at their school.

Though it may seem like a lot of work to hire an NP or a PA, it is *infinitely* less work to hire the right one than it is to hire the wrong one and go through the process again. In addition, it is important to note that most practices utilize at least one or two of the options listed above to obtain their NP or PA of choice. Other avenues are also possible, and those discussed may stimulate you to find other methods to reach the right candidate.

Effectively getting the word out is key to finding the right candidate. If you are patient and utilize multiple modalities, you may very well find the right candidate. There is a tremendous feeling when you find the person who fits your image for the position. The opportunity to work with and mentor the right candidate can make the process a wonderful experience.

Chapter 12
One Well-crafted E-mail
Causes the Cream to Rise

Initial Review and Prescreening Questions

If you are like me, you are familiar with the term "the cream rises to the top." It often refers to the fact that the best people somehow find a way to show why they are considered preeminent in their group. In hiring an NP or a PA, mechanisms are necessary to facilitate getting the optimal candidates to "rise to the top," which is what one well-crafted e-mail can do.

After you begin receiving cover letters and resumes from applicants, take the next step. Review the candidates' mailings and e-mails in batches once every week or two, to save time. Identify the NPs or PAs you feel are most highly suited for your practice.

Next, prescreen those outstanding candidates via an e-mailed list of questions like the following, which we use. You may select or withhold some of these questions, and/or use them at the in-person interview. The results will provide more insight into the people you are considering.

Notice that each step in the hiring process is designed to create a clearer picture of the candidate. The ideal scenario occurs when a few stand out so highly above the others that you can provide the next step to a more limited group.

The sample e-mail follows.

Name of Candidate: _____

Thank you for your interest in our position.

We have reviewed your cover letter and resume and would like to learn more about you. Several questions follow to help with this. Our goal is to have the best environment for our staff members and to have the best team in place. We appreciate your time and effort. Answer only the questions you are comfortable answering.

1. Are you currently employed? ___ Yes ___ No

2. Why are you leaving your current position, or why did you leave your most recent position?

3. If this is your first employment after graduation, why consider dermatology?

4. Do you have training in dermatology that would increase your value at hire? If so, explain.

5. If you do not have training in dermatology, be aware that dermatology is a highly intellectual field, requiring intense studying for eighteen to twenty-four months after being hired. What in your academic training shows your willingness to study and learn at this level?

6. Whether you do or do not have training in dermatology, what are you planning to do to attain proficiency, or greater proficiency, in dermatology?

7. Please list specific duties we can expect you to be proficient in, and, if you currently work, how many patients per day do you see (explain your job situation to us)?

8. What aspects of your educational process or prior jobs do/did you like?

9. Describe what aspects of your educational process or prior jobs you do/did not like.

10. Please list the strengths you see in yourself that we should know about.

11. What do you believe will make you stand out beyond other candidates?

12. What is your impression of the work you would do in a dermatology nurse practitioner or physician assistant capacity?

13. What do you see in an outpatient dermatology setting that makes you feel this could be your dream job?

14. How many days per week do you desire to work?
    ___ 5 days or 40 hours of patient care per week
    ___ 4 or fewer days per week (less than full time)
    ___ Either option is acceptable to me

15. Please describe the income you desire to make as a dermatology NP or PA.

16. What are your 5- and 10-year career goals?

17. Why would you consider this area to live?

Thank you for your time, and congratulations on being part of the upper tier of applicants. I look forward to getting to know you better.

Enthusiastically,

Roger T. Moore, MD

There may be other or additional questions you can ask that will help you identify the right candidate. For myself, it is helpful to know the type of dermatology work they have done, their level of commitment (including their plan for obtaining specialty knowledge), salary desired, and their long-term career goals.

The five- and ten-year goals are relevant to my future thinking and planning. As head of a practice who wants to mesh quality care with continuity, I use the response to this question to unmask future possibilities in the candidate, as well as future issues. One of my candidates indicated they wanted to be practicing in another location in five years. Finding that information at this stage of the hiring process was relevant to me.

As the person training the new hire, I also investigate how they respond to the questions about education. The candidates who appear willing to read on their own, and have a motivation or inquisitiveness about the conditions seen in clinic, are often the type who fit my style the best. Finding the right aptitude for learning in your candidate can be a significant factor.

As was the case for the resume and cover letter, these questions provide an opportunity for each candidate to communicate. You can see if their style of communication fits your practice. The professionalism, thoughtfulness, and articulation of ideas in the written word all give insight.

It may be easier to distinguish this when you get a group of respondents' questionnaires back and view them all at one time, but I have found that several typically stand out from the others in the application pool. From the top responders, you can begin to discern the finer points of the candidates.

The questions can be tailored to your desired investigative nature. Finding responses that identify the key factors you want to see in your NP or PA hire can add a layer of efficiency to the process of hiring.

Remember, the goal is to screen in a manner that outstanding candidates rise to the top with as little of your time required as possible. The e-mailed screening questions has been one of the best techniques to sort candidates that we have found, causing the cream to surge to the top.

Chapter 13
Conduct a High-yield
Phone Interview

Prepare a List of Fundamental Questions

After you have assessed the responses to your e-mailed questions, conduct telephone interviews of the top several candidates as the next step in the hiring sequence. Candidates who have dedicated the time to follow this sequence will view the practice as being organized, detail-oriented, and professional. This process is setting the tone and high standards expected for your future provider.

It is helpful to have a list of standard questions prepared and available to ask. The ability to compare candidates is essential and best done when they have each answered the same set of questions. Without a standardized method, evaluating between two candidates who are similar can be a challenge.

Here are a few ideas for questions, along with suggested interpretations to consider in the answers.

- What got you into the field you are working in now?
  - Favorable if the response meshes with your practice.
- Why are you leaving your current situation?
  - A response with excuses or blame may point to a less optimal outlook.
- Define your ideal job/position.
  - Responses that mesh with your position are expected, as most candidates prepare prior to the telephone interview. Instead, look for subtle clues that the candidate may be a good fit, such as an intellectual

nature, looking forward to the challenge of learning, or other qualities you are looking for.

- Do you have prior work or school experience you can share with me? (May need prompting.)
  - Be mindful for responses that mesh with the background you are looking for in a candidate.
- Why is this position of interest?
  - The response can give you insight into how much they have considered dermatology and what they have done to prepare for this opportunity.

Understand that each question asked should produce a response that can serve as an objective (not subjective) tool in your evaluation. This is the purpose of the phone call.

Plan to ask enough questions to determine whether the candidate may be a good fit for the practice. Make sure the person will mesh with the office's style and philosophy, and discover what they envision the job will be. Finding out expectations of a candidate can deter moving forward with a potential bad hire.

Prior to each phone interview, reread the candidate's resume as well as their responses to your e-mailed questions. Being familiar with the candidate will enable you to formulate new questions and identify any areas of concern you want to address. Add these new questions to your standard list. If you keyboard them into a word-processing document that you keep for that person, you will also be able to easily note their responses during the phone call.

When your questions have been prepared, pick up the telephone and call the candidate.

Techniques to Ensure an Efficient Interview

Your time is valuable, and a few techniques are necessary to make this an efficient use of your time and provide maximum results. The best results tend to occur with a "to the point" interview, which is brief and scripted.

Inform the candidate you are going to utilize a set of standard questions and it should only take a certain amount of time (i.e., fifteen minutes or less). Let them know you will be taking notes and this is the reason for any pauses. The candidates know they are being interviewed, so telling them you will be taking notes so you can remember them in the most positive light lets them know it is okay for a pause to occur.

Start the conversation with casual conversation. By establishing rapport, you create a more relaxed atmosphere for discussion, which allows for a smoother, quicker interview.

During the Call, Document and Rate the Responses

To administer the assessment, you can begin with introductory questions of your own that you feel will engage the candidate's professional interests and provide the means for you to further identity and connect with him or her.

Next, ask your standard questions, allow the candidate time to answer, and write your notes while they respond. If you waited until after the interview to write notes, you would extend the time you invest in the process. Do the note-taking during the call to be most efficient with your time.

It is essential to take enough notes that you can later recall how each interviewee responded. If you are writing or keyboarding and feel like the pause is becoming uncomfortable or a bit long, communicate that you are jotting down some notes.

Consider rating each response to your standard list of questions on a scale, 1 as low or unfavorable, and 3 as high or favorable. Then add up the points and see if the score corresponds to your intuitive feel about the candidate. If it is not, pause to identify the discrepancies.

The phone call with a number rating essentially provides you with an "NP or PA Candidate Assessment." This can be used in conjunction with the screening questions already received to further evaluate your top-scoring candidates.

Wrap up the phone call by describing how your office will be contacting them moving forward and the time line expected. Thank them for their time and you can ask if they have anything they would like to add or any questions.

The goal in this process is to efficiently continue to narrow down the candidate list to the best potential two or three candidates for your practice. The process described so far empowers you to focus your time on the highest yield candidates.

Again, remember that each step is designed to get useful, objective information, which in the end will help you make a sound decision in hiring your new provider.

Chapter 14
Create Your In-person Interview Assessment Guide

The face-to-face interview is a culmination of the screening tools already utilized. The time we will spend in person with a candidate will allow us to observe professionalism, personal interactions, and many intangibles. You are looking for a candidate who demonstrates the behaviors needed to be a success in your practice.

This is a time to focus on the fits and goals of your organization. Though some candidates possess a high likability factor, we must ensure this corresponds with the dedication, discipline, and determination needed to learn dermatology.

As physicians, we spend time daily with patients and often get a good feel for personality. However, the interview process is not something we do often, so setting objective parameters before the interview can be helpful.

As you did before the phone interview, prepare a standard set of questions for the in-person interview. This will make comparing different candidate's answers to the same questions easier. The subtle difference in answers can help delineate who may be the best fit.

A set of categories to consider rating candidates on is furnished below. You can tailor the list to your needs. Score each item, such as a 1 to 3 scale, then compile results after the interview.

Here are examples of behaviors that may be evaluated. Consider including these as you draft and organize interview questions to create your in-person interview assessment guide.

____ **Appearance:** Does the NP or PA dress appropriately and conduct themselves in a manner that matches your practice's and patients' expectations?

____ **Greeting:** Does the candidate present themselves with confidence and authority, as expected for a provider?

____ **Communication:** Do the exchanges with yourself, your staff, and patients appear engaging and appropriate for your office? (This is an area in which feedback from staff and others who interact with the NP or PA can also be valuable.)

____ **Listening skills:** Does the candidate ask clarifying questions, speak at appropriate times (not interrupt), maintain eye contact, nod or utilize other nonverbal tools to convey understanding, and engage in conversation fitting to the immediate situation?

____ **Social skills:** Does the candidate appear to establish rapport and interact well with others?

____ **Core values:** Are the in-person interactions and responses consistent with the responses given during prior assessments? (You might ask about a time they messed up and it was difficult to be honest with the boss/instructor/patient. How did they handle the situation?) (Look for other core values to determine whether they match your own professional values and those of your staff.)

____ **Dedication to learn the specialty:** Does the candidate provide information that displays they are committed to learning dermatology? (Plan to ask some questions to

ensure their desire to learn dermatology squares with
what has been stated so far. It is best to inquire what
books, journals, or other educational items they have
studied in the last six months. I ask, "What dermatology
resources do you currently have and use?" This can
unmask the person who states they have "a strong
desire" to do dermatology, from the person who is
actively working to expand their knowledge in
dermatology. I also ask, "What have you done to expand
your knowledge of dermatology?" This gives the
committed candidate an opportunity to shine. It can
reveal conferences attended, volunteer activities at
dermatology offices, journals read, and other ways they
have labored to improve their dermatology acumen. Or
it can result in a blank stare. Both are telling signs.)

____ **Coachability:** Does the candidate appear to take
direction well and be willing to follow your style of
practice? (Consider asking them to tell you about a time
they were encouraged to improve. Ask them in what
area. How did they respond to the request, and what was
the result? If they indicate they made a change in
themselves, improved future outcomes, and were
pleasant during the interaction, the coachability factor
might be high.)

____ **Time management/Organization:** Does the manner in
which they conduct themselves represent a person who
is organized and structured? (Asking questions of how
they structure their time, handle getting behind in clinic,
or manage stressful patients can be helpful.)

____ **Commitment to the practice:** Does the candidate
respond to questions in a way that indicates thinking
long-term with your practice? (In addition to finding out

about them and their dermatology knowledge, be absolutely certain to ask a few questions about their future. At times, they may flat out tell you they want their training so they can move to the wonderful place they have always dreamed of. This lets you know they plan to get the level of experience necessary to move on. Or they may tell you the location you are in is the one they always dreamed of and they want to stay forever. Though it is impossible to prevent a provider from gaining training and then leaving, the time invested in training on your part is best met with long-term thinking on the NP or PA's part.)

One standard question worth asking is, "What is the worst thing a previous employer would say about you?" This will be one of the times during the in-person interview you absolutely must be quiet and let the candidate answer. This is not the time to ease up and help them spin it off. It is a question to be answered honestly so that it provides needed insight.

When you write up the questions for the interview, consider including key administrative and medical staff members in the process, so that you will be sure to cover all your bases and conduct a thorough interview.

Be sure to outline the most important characteristics you are searching for. Creating a list of characteristics of the ideal candidate will help make it easier to select the candidate who most closely fits the bill.

Be aware that there are legal precedents to asking questions of candidates, and all your questions should be those accepted by state and local laws. There are questions an employer cannot ask. The guidelines are put into place to prevent employers from discriminating against potential hires.

To learn more about interview guidelines, find resources you trust. For our practice, the state chamber of commerce has been a wonderful resource. They provide a variety of services for businesses. In our state, there are books published with state-specific guidelines, including hiring, interviewing, and business practices. (The Indiana Chamber of Commerce, at www.indianachamber.com, has several books, including *Employment Law Handbook* by the law firm Faegre Baker Daniels, which we have found to be of particular value.)

A background check should also be run on your top candidate. Plan to ask applicants during the interview if they are under investigation, being audited by Medicare, or part of a pending liability litigation, as well as whether they have any convictions. If a candidate answers yes to any of those, it does not necessarily call for automatic elimination. If something like this comes up, it should be explored further. It is possible that a candidate may be part of a long list of physicians and NPs or PAs who provided care at some point to a patient who has filed a lawsuit. An audit does not always mean something is wrong. A candidate could possibly have gained unique experience and knowledge from such an experience that could benefit your practice. It is important to know about the situation and what the circumstances are.

The most important factor to keep in mind when drafting interview questions to separate out the right candidate is this: The person's personality and style must fit in with the practice and you as the supervising physician. You can hire the smartest or most qualified individual, though they must also be a good fit for the practice.

As with the phone interview, you'll need to beware of rehearsed responses. It is best to plan to ask questions and conduct the interview in a manner that gathers insight into strengths, weaknesses, and fit for the organization. Open-ended questions can provide insight beyond an expected answer. Ask questions to learn how they would handle situations. Do not be afraid to ask difficult questions.

The goal for the interview is to make the best possible decision for your practice. Having objective guides can facilitate a more accurate assessment. Prepare your own in-person interview assessment guide, from the questions you will ask to your parameters for scoring responses.

Through planning and creating this standardized assessment, you will gather objective data for the upcoming in-person interview, and you will provide yourself with a higher likelihood of selecting the optimal provider and ensuring ongoing practice success.

Chapter 15
Conduct a Revealing
In-person Interview

After you evaluate your phone interview notes, select your new top NP or PA candidates, and prepare your own in-person interview assessment guide, move to the next step in the hiring process—the in-person interview.

As you did prior to the phone interview, do your homework ahead of time. Know each candidate before they walk in the door. Review their cover letter, resume, their answers to your e-mailed questions, the notes you made when you spoke together on the phone, and how you scored them. Refresh your mind about their background so you do not waste valuable interview time asking questions that have already been answered in the paperwork. Then you can determine what still needs to be covered and focus on these questions as well as the assessment guide questions during the face-to-face interview.

There are any number of settings in which this interview can be conducted. The simplest method is to bring in the NP or PA for a one-on-one session. If this sit-down convinces you they are worthy of further consideration, following it with a dinner afterward can be useful.

This provides an opportunity to have a structured and reproducible interview session followed by a more relaxed session. The dinner is often the "get to know you" phase, when you learn more about a candidate personally. The armor or shield most people put up for the interview is lowered, and you may connect more authentically.

Another method I like includes adding some time for the NP or PA to shadow me at the office. Sharing a day or partial day at the office provides invaluable insight. This can occur not only with physician/candidate interaction but also staff, patients, and other NP or PAs (if you have them). While the candidate interacts with patients, you can see a bit more about whether the personality fits your style. Though you can't learn everything about a person during shadowing, you can often get a general feel. After the candidate leaves, you might also request feedback from others in the office who may have noted interactions you were not privy to.

We opt for a combination approach. We ask the candidate to come in for a few hours to see how the practice operates, meet the staff, and shadow in the office. This gives the dermatologist and the entire staff a sense of their professionalism, demeanor, and ability to interact with staff and patients. After this a formal sit-down interview is conducted with structured questions. The dinner setting is often reserved for the highest potential candidates or those coming in from out of town.

One time we had a candidate who gave a smooth phone interview and seemed like a great fit. During the shadowing process, he continued to share his knowledge, or lack thereof, to patients repeatedly. He seemed to thrive on being a know-it-all. The icing on the cake was when a patient had benign lesions on the skin examination that I was explaining, and he rolled up his sleeves, interrupted, and shared with the patient that he had those same lesions and she should not worry. Though his interaction might not have bothered some physicians, his in-person antics and interruption did not mesh well with what I wanted in our candidate.

You want someone you are willing to teach and enjoy sharing your knowledge with. Your efforts for this person should create a feeling of accomplishment as you see them find their way and succeed. The personality component of your evaluation is instrumental here since you will spend quite a bit of time together.

Through the process of hiring, you are, in essence, selling your practice environment and yourself to the candidate. At the same time, and more importantly, the candidate is working to sell him- or herself to you as the best fit for your organization.

At the end of this shadowing session, take time to ask the questions from your interview assessment guide, plus any other questions that have not been answered.

Throughout the interview, do not intervene too soon when silence occurs.

Following are other helpful tips for the interviewing process.

- **Remember the personal element.** While it is important to get answers to medical-specific questions, it is also important to get to know the candidate on a personal level. Use your questions as a template, but be sure to listen to what your candidate is saying and be willing to go in a different direction. It can be helpful to chat with them about their life outside of medicine. Find out what inspires them and what they enjoy doing. Remember, finding a candidate that meshes well in terms of personality is a key to hiring the individual.

- **Do not accept general answers.** Dig deeper to find out what the candidate knows and what they think by listening to what they say and allowing the conversation to take on its own nature, at times directed by the candidate. It is too easy to avoid the specifics, and on a day-to-day basis, those can be points of contention. Draw out of them the items you feel are important (i.e., support staff expected, time willing to devote to education, limitations expected, call expectations, what they expect from you for training, how committed they are to your practice, etc.).

- **Do not rely on memory.** When you are interviewing several candidates, take notes during each interview so that later you will be able to remember what each candidate had to say. Accurately recalling details can be important in decision-making.

Wrap up the interview by giving them three minutes to share why they would be the best candidate for your position.

Once the interview is over, let the candidate know where they stand and what they should expect next. When will they hear from you next? How much longer will you be conducting interviews? Always follow up. Remember that you are dealing with a person's livelihood, so make sure to be respectful and handle interviews in a timely manner.

After the Interview, Be Sure to Check References

For a hire of this magnitude, it is imperative that you contact the references!!! You might be tempted to skip this step, but following through can yield astute insight you might not otherwise attain.

This should not be delegated for this level of hire. Check references personally. Ask if your candidate would be eligible for rehire. An answer in the positive will reveal that they left or are leaving on good terms, while an answer in the negative means you likely need to gain more information about the candidate.

Creating a brief list of standardized questions to ask the references can be helpful. Look to identify strong traits, deficiencies, and areas of concern. A question I have found helpful is asking, "How does [the candidate] compare with others you have worked with?" Give a scale to the person you are speaking with, such as "average," or "in the fiftieth percentile," "the top 25 percent" they have worked with, or one of the best they have worked with, such as, "the top 10 percent." Answers to the rating of a candidate can sometimes verify or contradict the results you have gained so far in your interview process.

Remember that the goal of the interview and hiring process is to attain information and to identify whether the person is a great fit for your organization. Acquiring thorough and consistent data can help guide your decision-making process.

Chapter 16
These Five Traits:
The Ultimate Secret to Hiring the
Right Candidate

The Immeasurable Worth Teamwork

Some of the most successful businesspeople in my area have said that it is "*all* in the people." The CEOs and owners give credit to the people who work with and for them. The president of one such company, Mr. Clark, and his two partners sold their RV company for over $500 million dollars before it was ten years old. When I asked him how he did it, he shared that it is all in the people you bring onto your team.

His company had actually won a national award for entrepreneurial spirit the year before they sold their business. When I read details about it in the newspaper, he described that he was so proud and appreciative of the entire group of employees that he had a T-shirt printed up with the company name and award they won on the front. On the back, he listed every single employee's name—in tiny print, but every name was there.

To him, each employee mattered to the organization and its success. The morale he orchestrated helped make him wealthy, and at the same time made each person on the team feel great about being there.

So teamwork is one non-negotiable trait that a top candidate must possess.

Empathy: A Leading Tenet of Success

Having empathy is also essential to success. Empathy is the ability to feel what another person feels, and thus it helps a person relate to others in similar situations.

I did not fully appreciate this until our daughter, in eighth grade, had surgery on her knee for a tear in her articular cartilage. The orthopedic surgeon and his staff were kind, but they did not give us therapy orders the day of surgery, so no therapy was provided.

Her knee just did not seem to be healing right. She would not let anyone touch her knee because it hurt her so badly, and she remained on crutches. Three weeks later we called the surgeon's office. Unfortunately, the doctor had left town after her surgery to attend the NFL draft combine for a few weeks, and now was on a family vacation for another week. As parents we felt a great deal of anxiety.

We placed more phone calls, and the medical assistant finally arranged for therapy.

Though it seemed like an eternity, we finally made it to the four-week follow-up. The orthopedic surgeon spent just a minute or two looking at her (she would not let him do much with the knee) and asking a couple of questions. He said she had reflex sympathetic dystrophy. Then he asked if she had any questions.

My shy daughter looked up and asked, "When will I be able to feel and move my foot?"

He retorted that would be up to her, that she had to work on it as he had done his part. Then he stood up in his white coat and left the room. The surgeon did not mention a follow-up to us on his way out.

At that moment, my heart sunk as a parent. We watched the person we felt would hold answers and solutions dart in with a proclamation, a tip or two on the treatment, and then leave.

Suddenly, I thought back to how many people have come into my office wanting an answer only to leave without one. And worse yet, how many have left with the belief that I didn't want to see them back since I didn't mention a follow-up.

I left that day never wanting to give the feeling that I had received to any patient of mine. Now I most certainly do not want to think his cavalier approach was intended to cause emotional distress. At the same time, as I watched my daughter deflate like the air had been let out of her, I did conclude we as providers should never lose our empathy.

That moment was a turning point for me. With all the pressures of health care that we experience as providers, the one constant is that our patients want to feel like someone is on their side.

So, the very least a person can do as a health care provider is to reassure each patient that they are there for them and will do their best to see them through the problem they have. No matter how hard the path is, being there for them, or putting them in the hands of someone who will be there for them (as in a referral to someone else), is important to do.

When the days seem too busy to be there and mean it, then we need to reset and intentionally think about the patient. When we do this, we will help our patients, and by default help the practice.

Hiring for Teamwork and Empathy

When hiring (and training) your new NP or PA, be certain that they believe patient care, specifically empathy, is always of the utmost importance, as is genuine teamwork among the staff.

Having a staff and providers who put each patient and their problem first is one of the cornerstones of building a successful business. As the leaders of our practices, we must live this point, and teach it. In the hiring process, when you pick a person who will walk this path with you, the rewards will be multiplied in referrals alone.

Once I determine that a candidate's personality and experience are a good fit for our practice, the three additional factors I have found most important in determining eligibility are these.

1. **Willingness to learn/education acumen:** The candidate must have a full understanding there are high expectations placed on them to learn not only in clinic, but also in their time outside of the office. The best candidates will commit to mastering the specialty and take ownership of a significant portion of their own educational process.

2. **Commitment to patients (obligation to doing their job well):** This is the person who is willing not only to look up conditions for the patient, but also is willing to call the patient with results.

3. **Longevity in practice (someone who is looking to stay long-term):** Though this can never be predicted, I make note of any comments made that suggest the true future plans of the NP or PA. The time I dedicate to educating an NP or a PA is so involved, that in my opinion the person who wants to work a year and then move is best to learn from someone else. Consider asking questions like these. "What are your five-year goals?" Or, "Paint a picture of your professional life in five or ten years."

When you are ready to make the decision, consider obtaining input from key administrative and medical support staff, because they too will be working with this individual and may have different impressions than you do.

Be sure to follow up and provide closure to every candidate interviewed. The values of empathy and consideration for others extend to them. In addition, you never know when your paths might cross again, and those you interviewed can be future referring providers.

Keep in mind that the art of finding the right person is like the art of medicine. You can do the very best to be as prepared as possible, and even with a great deal of preparation end up in a tough situation. Each step in the hiring process is done to help maximize a positive outcome for you and your candidates.

In general, a well-thought-out and -organized interview process can lead to the best hire. Almost equally important is that the best candidates are attracted by structure and professionalism. The joy of having the right NP or PA can truly add value to the practice for your patients and light a brighter fire in yourself and your staff. The time you invest in this part of the process can pay dividends many times over for your future.

Chapter 17
Understand Credentialing
and Privileging

Once you have narrowed down the list of candidates, before extending an offer, check on the candidate's credentials to make certain they are properly educated and licensed. Much of this information can be obtained online from the state professional licensing agency.

In addition, the American Academy of Nurse Practitioners Certification Board has a website (www.aanpcert.org) where you can verify national certification.

The National Commission on Certification of Physician Assistants also has a website (www.nccpa.net) where physician assistant certification can be confirmed.

The American Medical Association website provides a tool that allows you to verify a physician assistant candidate's legal name, date of birth, address, education, graduation, national certification status, and current and past state licensure information at the American Medical Association Physician Profile (https://commerce.ama-assn.org/amaprofiles/).

During the hiring process, perhaps after a second interview (or third, if three are needed), you should request the following documentation from each candidate who is considered. (Always be sure to check the expiration dates on all licenses and certifications.)

> ➢ A copy of his or her current state license. This should include their license number, DEA number (if applicable), and expiration dates.

> A copy of current certification from the National Commission on Certification of Physician Assistants (NCCPA) for PAs, or a copy of current certification from either the American Academy of Nurse Practitioners (AANP) or the American Nurses Credentialing Center (ANCC) for NPs.
> Letters of recommendation from previous employers and colleagues that include evaluation of the performance of specific responsibilities.
> Documentation of Continued Medical Education (CME) records or any additional training the provider has received.
> A copy of any recent hospital privileges, and a log that documents specific procedures performed (if applicable).

Though not entirely related to the credentialing of a provider, the process of how an NP or a PA can bill is worth understanding, since it pertains to the economics after hiring. The items worth reviewing during this section are the "direct" and "incident-to" billing for the NP or PA. As mentioned earlier in the book, Medicare reimburses for NP or PA services at 85 percent the rate of the physician fee schedule. This is when the NP or PA is utilizing "direct billing," meaning they are the provider who initiates care and responsibility for the patient and the diagnosis the patient is seen for.

A bill can also be rendered for services provided by an NP or a PA as "incident-to," which is reimbursed at the physician's fee schedule when certain parameters are met. This is a topic I recommend you go the Centers for Medicare and Medicaid Services (CMS) website and research to understand fully. The information presented here is not legal advice but only a generalization of my own interpretation/summary from the CMS

article from MLM Matters Numbers SE0441
(https://www.cms.gov/Outreach-and-Education/Medicare-Learning-Network-MLN/MLNMattersArticles/downloads/se0441.pdf).

The article from the CMS website states the following. "To qualify as "incident-to," services must be part of your patient's normal course of treatment, during which a physician personally performed an initial service and remains actively involved in the course of treatment. You do not have to be physically present in the patient's treatment room while these services are provided, but you must provide direct supervision, that is, you must be present in the office suite to render assistance, if necessary. The patient record should document the essential requirements for incident-to service."

The entire article is worth reading so that you fully understand the rules and guidelines of "incident-to" billing. The economic advantage can be significant, if the visit qualifies for the physician's fee schedule.

Chapter 18
Getting a Basis for What Salary
Is Expected by Candidates

Does a Formula Exist to Calculate Wages for the NP or PA?

Typically, physicians do not want to put much more than cursory effort into determining an NP or a PA's wages. However, for many candidates, the expected salary is a big factor in their selecting the specialty they plan to go into. They often have this tabbed as their first consideration. They know the expected salary before they ever start submitting applications.

This is not all bad, as compensation is a driving force for many adults in their employment, including the field they choose to enter. But it is important for the physician to keep abreast of current salary information, trends, and how NPs or PAs are paid.

It is important to put time into this, including a rationale for the pay scale you will set. This research should be one of the early steps in the planning and hiring process, as noted in Chapter 4.

A variety of methods for remuneration are available for NPs and PAs. Though there is not a wrong or right answer to what amount you are going to pay, the golden nugget is that the contract needs to be competitive in the marketplace. In most cases the new hire will have wandering eyes as soon as they sign with you, and no matter how much training and time is invested on your end, if a situation opens up that is more enticing (specifically, more profitable), you may lose your NP or PA.

Tracking down the market salary can be like trying to hold onto a slippery fish. It seems to never stay in the same location, and when you think you have it caught, a slight move can cause a rapid change, making you lose your grip on the situation.

For the pay of an NP or a PA to remain competitive, you must establish good communication, build trust, and maintain an eye on the current market.

There is not a single published formula to best calculate pay. The key is to develop a model that provides your practice with something you feel comfortable to offer and, at the same time, the NP or PA believes is a good deal for them. When both parties feel they have a fair situation, the likelihood of a long-lasting relationship is greater.

Guidelines

In many instances, the first year (or early years) of practice in a specific specialty are salary based. Salaries vary, depending upon geographic location, community size, and the duties that will be performed.

After the practitioner obtains proficiency in the specialty, incentives are often incorporated. Basis for bonus can vary greatly, with common platforms being the following.

- money brought into the practice (i.e., percentage of collections)
- number of patients seen
- other measurable parameters utilized for some or all of the bonus or incentive package

Two common models of payment are low-base and high-base pay. Both are tied to benefits for the provider and the practice.

Usually the low base has an enticing productivity scale to it (less reassurance of the higher income). The productivity bonus can outweigh the low-base pay/salary if a provider is diligent and efficient at seeing patients. This provides the practice lower risk since the NP or PA must work to attain the bonus.

The high-base pay model also usually has a productivity bonus, though it can be less in some form than the low-base pay model. The practice takes on more of a risk with the higher base pay model, while the NP or PA obviously takes on less risk. The new hire also has more security in knowledge of their annual salary at the outset.

The NP or PA is often paid the salary biweekly or monthly, and then the bonus is distributed quarterly, semiannually, or annually.

In most states, NPs and PAs are exempt, as opposed to nonexempt (hourly wage workers), from the overtime rules since they are classified as "professionals." This is similar to physicians and does not require payment for time outside the normal forty-hour work week (such as charting, patient callbacks, and the like).

What Approximate Salary Do Candidates Expect?

The first step to learning what the market is for NPs and PAs nationally is to look through salary websites, national associations, nurse practitioner or physician assistant societies, and the Bureau of Labor Statistics. Associations such as the American Academy of Nurse Practitioners and the American Academy of Physician Assistants also tend to have general information available or links to relevant websites.

However, these numbers may lag behind the more real-time numbers, because some of the surveys are done only every several years. Also, since these estimations may not be for specific specialties, it may take more effort to find what the market is for a specialty such as dermatology. Finding a more accurate salary range for your region, your size and type of practice, among other factors might take a bit more effort. Local estimates can be found on job search engines, but less information about data used to compile the surveys is available.

Specialty organizations such as Society of Dermatology Physician Assistants (SDPA) do perform surveys of salaries at times, as well. One of the helpful aspects of past SDPA surveys is the inclusion of statistics and categories for different regions, specific subspecialties, and years of experience. All of these are important factors in determining wages when hiring.

In addition, medical societies and professional organizations can be great resources for determining salary ranges and benefits for NP and PA candidates. The Society of Dermatology Physician Assistants (www.dermpa.org) has had salary surveys in the past, with subcategories such as academic affiliation, years of experience, geographic location, and other groupings. Likewise, the Medical Group Management Association (www.mgma.com) has a salary survey, one that is used by many larger health care systems.

A small amount of time spent researching these websites will help you approximate the salary of NPs and PAs in your region.

Consider also talking to the human resources department of the hospital you have credentials with, as they are often in tune with the current market. Hospital systems do not compete with dermatology services in many areas and may be willing to provide information. The hospitals routinely use the MGMA data and might be able to provide you some reference points from survey results they have access to. The hospitals or area multispecialty groups can also provide information as to the typical compensation package for primary care NP and PAs, which can give a reference point.

Recruiters of dermatology professionals may also be quite helpful in providing the trends of what they see as possible pay structures. Leaders or officers of the state or national dermatology societies for NPs or PAs may provide information or offer names of other dermatologists in your state who might be willing to share information.

In one of our hiring cycles, I contacted a past president of the SDPA who was more than willing to share trends, current models, and basic parameters of compensation. The data was helpful, and I found having an officer of the respected SDPA organization provide information reassuring. Part of the commitment of the society office, whether it is local, regional, or national, is to help forward the specialty, and your willingness to seek input from them is often welcomed and appreciated.

Even if you are a small practice, you want to be aware of the market and compensation for regional NP or PA providers so you can choose the best compensation package for your situation.

A variety of factors besides pay and bonus are considerations in the structure of a contract, including benefits such as health insurance, retirement plan, CME allowance, malpractice coverage, and vacation time. The MGMA and other salary surveys described above can help give an idea of the amount of each of these items.

Some salary structures described in the following chapter provide a general idea. They are not meant to be set in stone or used as legal documentation but rather tools to explore.

Chapter 19
How to Create Your Own
Payment Model

A Word about Ballpark Numbers

The base pay varies quite a bit. Some practices offer at or below $70,000, while others compensate at or above $120,000. On multiple occasions, I have encountered new graduates from NP and PA schools wanting to get into the field who have viewed their desired salary as that "posted" for the specialty. For example, as of this writing, the AANP website student resource center tab "starting your career" indicated that new NPs had an average annual total income reported to be $91,060. We had several responses to an ad for a new NP or PA where the applicants—some new graduates with no experience, and some with family practice or hospital experience—requested base pay of over $100,000. (It is worth mentioning that none of the candidates had done so much as a dermatology rotation or any other dermatology experience.)

One stated the current rate published for dermatology was $100,000, and this was the rationale for wanting the starting salary she requested. The mind-set was that the average dermatology NP or PA made that rate, and thus they wanted to begin with that.

Unfortunately, it is hard to rationalize paying the average base pay to a new graduate who will take a minimum of months to attain any level of proficiency. It might also be worth asking why they request the amount they do. At times, you might find the area hospitals or other clinics are offering an amount higher than you expected. It may impact how you structure an agreement.

One of my NPs, when renewing his contract, suggested pay in the $200,000 range. I was a bit taken aback at first and asked why he thought this. He brought in a survey of dermatology NPs that showed the mean income was $199,000 per year. This survey had come from an Internet source neither of us had heard of before. The site's survey included six participants but very little distinguishing information. There were no regions of the country, number of patients seen, hours worked, surgical procedures, or other data to review and understand the origin of the high pay. It was hard to determine how it compared to the workload and type of work we asked of our NPs.

Sample Salary Structures

For new graduates or those new to the field of dermatology, a reasonable approach is to have only base pay (no other financial incentive) for the first six to twelve months. This is due in part to the time the supervising physician invests training while the NP or PA shadows and learns. For a full-time NP or PA (seeing patients/shadowing the physician 36 to 40 hours per week), the base pay can range from $70,000 to $90,000 per year, depending, in part, upon location.

During this first year, the NP or PA will gain knowledge of the specialty and establish rapport with patients and staff. The amount of supervision is typically significant, and independent contact with patients much lower, than is the case for an established provider with strong knowledge of dermatology.

If an NP or a PA has moderate to extensive experience, a base salary plus a percentage of collections after a certain threshold is common. The practice must discern what is a good fit, based on the overhead (direct and indirect costs of the NP or PA's practice).

It may be easier to think of salary and bonus on an annual basis, but the payments of bonuses can be calculated at a time interval convenient for you and practice. It is not uncommon for the bonus structures to be allocated quarterly, biannually, or annually.

Several examples of methods to pay the NP or PA can be employed. A few will be shared here. The information is not meant to be legal advice, but rather conceptual ideas to help build your own pay structure. It is recommended you consult a health care attorney to review your contract, especially compensation. This is an area where there should be no ambiguity. Fairness to both the practice and the NP or PA is essential and accomplished by a lawyer's well-written contract.

For simplicity's sake, we will discuss numbers in an annual format from here forward.

Straight Percentage Method of Pay

If a provider joined your group and was paid only a percentage of collections, the computations would be easy. For instance, if the NP or PA in your practice brought in total net collections (net receipts/collected revenue) at the end of the year of $500,000, then this number would be used to form calculations. If they were to get 20 percent of the total year's net collections, their pay would be 20 percent of $500,000, which equals $100,000.

The percentage of total collections that practices use when computing in this manner can vary from 20 percent to as high as 35 percent. The variation in percentage can be tied to any number of factors, such as the following.

- experience

- collection threshold reached
- number of patients seen
- surgical procedures performed
- cosmetic treatments rendered
- alternative expenses
- base salary

and more.

A common variant of this is the NP or PA is provided a base salary and then, at specified time intervals, the total net collections are reviewed to determine if the provider has earned a productivity bonus.

An example might be a contract that stipulates the NP or PA has a base salary of $80,000 and is eligible to receive the base pay or to be paid 20 percent of year-end net collections—if that amount is greater than base pay.

- In this scenario, if the NP or PA who was hired with a base salary of $80,000 and was to get base salary or 20 percent of collections at year end (whichever was greater), where year-end total net collections were $500,000, then the provider would get a $20,000 bonus. The $20,000 bonus is because 20 percent of the $500,000 equals $100,000. This would bring the total compensation to $100,000, since it is greater than the base pay.
- If that same provider only brought in year-end total net collections of $300,000, there would be no bonus, since 20 percent of $300,000 is $60,000, and thus less than base pay.

Double Base Pay + Bonus

Another method involves doubling the base pay and providing a productivity bonus on total net collections above the doubled base pay amount. Thus, a bonus (typically 5 to 10 percent of his or her total net collections) is given after two times the base salary is reached.

Again, determining the bonus percentage is practice-specific, in part due to the variabilities in practice and in the provider's style of practice, overhead, and experience.

An example of this method of bonus pay appears in the following scenario, for a provider with a base salary of $85,000.

Once double the base salary amount has been earned—$170,000 in net collections—then the NP or PA is eligible for a bonus.

For instance, if the NP or PA has net collections of $300,000 in a year . . .

$300,000 minus $170,00 = $130,000
$130,000 times 10 percent = **$13,000 bonus**

The total pay for the year would be . . .

$85,000 (base pay) + $13,000 (bonus) = **$98,000**

The percentage for the productivity bonus can vary and must fit what you are comfortable paying.

The productivity bonus, and the corresponding percentage rate it is placed at, is based on varied factors such as the following.

- experience
- number of surgical or cosmetic procedures performed
- amount of supervision by physician
- working in independent sites/clinic locations
- administrative duties/management of staff
- amount of other benefits the NP or PA receives as part of his or her compensation

Some practices have increased the amount of percentage to as high as 30 to 35 percent when the NP or PA is very experienced, has a full patient schedule, and performs duties that generate sufficient revenue for the practice to justify this percentage.

Some practices include in the computation of base pay *all direct costs* for the NP or PA. This includes his or her employee benefits plus monies paid out for having the provider work at the practice. For example:

- $7200/year health care
- $6000/year—payroll taxes
- $1000/year—malpractice insurance
- $1800/year—continuing education

That is an additional $16,000 per year of direct costs. This $16,000 is added to the $85,000 base pay before computing bonuses.

In this scenario, the NP or PA would have a base pay of $101,000 ($85,000 + $16,000 = $101,000), which must be doubled in order to become eligible for the productivity bonus. Once the NP or PA becomes eligible, he or she would get 10 percent of net collections over $202,000 as their bonus for the year.

Tiered Percentage for Pay

A tiered percentage is also a method that can be beneficial for the practice and the NP or PA. In this setting, an NP or a PA will get a low percentage after the threshold amount, and the percentage can be increased for the dollars earned after a higher threshold.

For example, after net collections of 2 times base + direct costs, the NP or PA receives a bonus of 5 percent of net collections for the first $500,000 of total collections (be aware: it is money *collected*, not charges). Then, after net collections of $500,000, the bonus percentage on each dollar goes up to 10 percent. This way, the NP or PA is incentivized to hit the threshold mark, and the stability of the practice is bolstered through their work.

In 2017, the Society of Dermatology Physician Assistants placed on its website (www.hireadermpa.com/compensation-benefits.com) similar information to that presented above, though with less detail. It also suggested that in an "ideal" setting the PA would get 33 percent of net collections, while 33 percent would go to overhead costs and 33 percent would go to the supervising physician. Unfortunately, the overhead percentage is antiquated in this scenario for most practices, as the changes in health care have all but eliminated the possibility of overhead being as low as 33 percent for a provider.

In our practice, a PA left after two years of what I considered very diligent training and investment of my own time and our team's effort to train him. It was disheartening to lose the PA, who left for a higher base pay and same percentage of collections, when in all likelihood at the end of the year he would have had the same pay. It reminded me that I would like it to be difficult financially for a good PA to leave and find a comparable job. This philosophy may not fit every physician, but for me it fits with geographic location, overhead, and style of practice.

One point to consider, if you elect to do any time interval less than one year, is to incorporate some equalizing factors for vacation. We had a PA take most of the vacation in one quarter and then the next quarter had high volume and corresponding charges. In a quarterly productivity mode, you can imagine what happened. The PA was considerably below the "productivity threshold" in one quarter and significantly above it in the next. It is therefore advisable to think about the potential fluctuations in patient volume, and thus total net collections can vary with vacation and time of year. It is best to make sure your health care attorney writes the contract to account for these variables.

As mentioned before, there is no single way to determine compensation and benefits. The practical point is to know what risk your practice is willing to support. Be aware of the regional and/or national market compensation scale, and also evaluate overhead. Tie all of this knowledge together and create a payment model that reflects the current medical climate and their practices. With good communication with your NP or PA candidates, you can then form a team that will grow your practice together long-term.

For More Information . . .

Though there are not a lot of set standards, the following articles outline a few considerations in addition to those described above.

- "Use objective measures to incentivize mid-level providers for increased productivity." *Medical Economics.* April 8, 2014. Debra Phairas. http://medicaleconomics.modernmedicine.com/medical-economics/content/tags/incentive/use-objective-measures-incentivize-midlevel-providers-incre?page=0,1
- "The PA Salary: Structures and Strategies." *Practical Dermatology.* August 2012. Katherine Wilkens, PA-C, MHIS, MPAP. http://practicaldermatology.com/2012/08/the-pa-salary-structures-and-strategies/

Chapter 20
Ways to Take the Fear out of Investing in the NP or PA

At times, the thought of investing upward of $100,000 in a person who has no dermatology experience can be daunting. Some techniques I use to provide physicians some comfort in their situations are worth mentioning here. These are ideas to help alleviate the fear of investing a great deal of time, money, and resources into someone who might not work out. There is no right or wrong approach. Decide which strategies best fit you and your practice.

First three months at half pay. During the interview process, one of my colleagues conveys to top candidates who have no dermatology experience that the first 90 days will be the NP or PA's time to learn, show their merit, and find ways to help grow the practice. For these first three months, the new NP or PA will be paid at half the monthly rate of the rest of the year's pay. After month three, my colleague will pay the new NP or PA a fair market monthly salary. The colleague feels this is fair, as do the candidates.

Educational compensation agreement. If hiring a new provider to the specialty, an option for him or her to cover expenses and time invested in training can be incorporated into an educational compensation agreement. Though this can have many variables, a consideration is to place a dollar amount on the value of the physician's time, with an estimate of how much is going to be invested in training or education for the first year or so. A dollar amount both the NP or PA and supervising physician agree is reasonable can be entered in the agreement. The thrust of this point is that the NP or PA will repay this expense if they leave the practice soon after the physician has fully trained them and ensured that they are proficient in the specialty. If the NP or PA leaves partway through the training, they compensate the physician a prorated amount. The NP or PA can find this acceptable, since, if they choose to leave, they will have the potential to be in a higher earning specialty for the remainder of their career.

Restrictive covenants. There is debate about the legality of a restrictive covenants (aka non-compete clause, or NCC) in some states. Reasonableness and needs in the community seem to play a factor in several of the debates. Still it is not uncommon to have them placed in providers' agreements. Most contract lawyers in the state of the practice should be familiar with restrictions and have recommendations in this realm.

To think something is not needed may be fine with some practices, while with others it is not. Changes can happen for a variety of reasons and at times cannot be prevented. It is best to ease your fears and safeguard your investment and practice by making use of the above, and/or similar, strategies.

Chapter 21
What Should Be Included in the Employment Contract?

When you make your decision to hire, you will then be ready to extend an offer to your candidate. This includes having a contract drawn up that complies with all state practice laws and regulations. The contract should also clearly lay out the relationship you expect the new provider to have with the supervising physician and the staff. It is best to seek advice from a lawyer who is familiar with the regulations of your state.

For most entities, the clauses included can be standard. However, tailoring the contract is largely on your shoulders. If you would like an educational compensation agreement or a restrictive covenant placed in your agreement, it is something you will need to have your lawyer collaborate on.

I have personally found it works best to have the lawyer supply me with a contract, and then I write them a note or e-mail detailing what is to be added. The legal team then takes the contract and amends it to make it appropriate.

A **restrictive covenant** clause to add might be if your local area has many medical spas or surgery centers that market themselves as skin cancer institutes but are run by non-dermatologists. You can ask your lawyer about the viability of including a restriction that prevents your NP or PA from working at one of these institutes in a manner that competes with you after you train him or her. The lawyer can then determine if restrictions of the sort are appropriate and/or worthwhile to place in the contract.

Malpractice insurance guidelines should be included in the contract. Most practices will pay for the malpractice coverage of the NP or PA. This should always be addressed in the employment contract to ensure appropriate coverage. Areas that should be addressed include the following.

- payment of the premium by the practice (or the NP or PA)
  - In addition, a clause is typically present that indicates the provider must be eligible for malpractice to continue employment.
- type of coverage—Insurance terms should also be referenced in the collaborative agreement to ensure there is appropriate coverage for all areas where the NP or PA will be providing patient care on behalf of your practice. Ask the malpractice carrier if the coverage is "claims made coverage" or requires a "tail" for the NP or PA if they leave the practice.
- claims that might be made for actions that took place during previous employment
- which party is responsible for malpractice coverage (especially if a "tail" is required to be purchased) upon termination or expiration of the employment agreement

Separation factors should be placed in the contract. This would include items such as how to handle net collections, bonus payments, CME, vacation days, and so on, in the event the NP or PA leaves your practice. It would certainly not make a practice feel as though they were treated fairly if CME and vacation days for a year were used and then the NP or PA left only a third of the way through the contract year. Thus, having guidelines for separation on prorated vacation days, CME days, and how to handle bonus payments, and the like, are best included in the initial agreement.

Though there are any number of details in a contract, it is best to take time to iron them out before any issues can arise. A solid contract that irons out the ambiguities provides a guideline for the practice and the provider.

Part Three

Training and Education

Chapter 22
You, the Mentor

When we think about training our NPs and PAs, we should consider our impact. The mannerisms you show to them, the staff, and the patients are what you are encouraging them to do by default. We must focus on how we want our patients treated and cared for.

It is worth reminding ourselves as physicians, *As you go, so goes your team.* A can-do attitude and servant mentality by "the doctor" will set a tone and establish a positive culture. The rest of the team members around you will reflect you—in their tone of voice to patients, their words spoken, their mannerisms. And if you don't believe this, listen to how your medical assistants call a few patients back. Whatever they say will often sound eerily similar to what you say in the exam room, including voice inflection. Try it.

Gandhi was credited with the quote, "Be the change you want to see in the world." Though we may not change the world, if we make sure we are representing who we would like our staff to be, we can make a larger impact than we imagine.

As you think of yourself as a mentor, keep in mind that the NP or PA you train is apt to have minuscule to no knowledge of our specialty, just as you once possessed no specialized knowledge. This means they are so dependent on your guidance now, that it is as though they are walking in the dark, and you are holding a lantern, directing them each step of the way.

Therefore, you must assume the role of mentor. The mentor can help light a dark path for a person who has yet to travel in the same direction. Set the example of what you expect them to be, within the confines of their own personality, of course. Each physician must represent the person they would like their NP or PA to be in the approach to patient care, handling of staff, and academic interlay.

Unfortunately, we physicians can get jaded by the changes in health care and find cynicism a method of handling the uneasy feeling that comes with forced change. The repeated attacks, burdens, and stresses placed squarely on the shoulders of physicians can reduce our occupation to a job. Most providers entered the field of medicine to have a profession of caring and compassion with a byproduct of being well compensated. The upheaval in government regulations, practice dynamic changes, and so much more can change our thinking and alter our ability to be the mentor and role model our team needs.

Think back to childhood, when most of us looked up to one or more people we admired who exemplified traits we could envision ourselves emulating, such as parents, teachers, coaches, and even sports heroes, musicians, or movie stars. As we grew older, we became more independent in our thinking as we each evolved into our own person. Today, as adult goal-oriented, type A personalities, most of us physicians have developed a sense of idealism based on combined experiences of ourselves, our interactions with the world around us, and the people we interact with or see take action. At the same time, we still find people we draw inspiration from. Many of these life experiences and people we interact with continue to shape who we are and how we live and practice.

What is it that inspires you about your mentors? Is it their energy, enthusiasm, dedication, intellectual prowess, or some other attribute? If you can identify one or more traits your mentors have provided to you, strive to exemplify them to your NP or PA.

A mentor can become a guiding beacon that shapes a career for many years to come. Many of the people placed in the path of a training physician can take on a role of displaying some of the most wonderful and powerful attributes of human nature in dealing with patients, staff members, and other professionals. These mentees may gradually become mentors to others through their actions.

A true mentor, though, is someone who goes a step beyond setting the example. He or she intentionally shepherds and guides another provider, being a resource for continued growth, an encourager, and a person who holds someone accountable on their road to success.

If you have not done so, consider taking the time to pinpoint several attributes you want to mentor for your NP or PA. What do you want represented when another add-on is placed on the schedule? What interaction with patients do you want when you are an hour behind? What do you want done when medical assistant does not think ahead in the exam room?

Remember that a calm smile and "we can do it" attitude by the leader can trickle down fast.

When you consciously mentor the qualities you admire, you create the culture that you want all of your team members to emulate and your patients to experience . . . and to look forward to experiencing again.

Chapter 23
Engendering Trust

To you and your patients, and for you and your NP or PA, trust matters.

The quality of education received by an NP or a PA can be observed by the patients. In fact, it is often more transparent than even the physician, NP, or PA can imagine. Patients see right through the provider who learns nothing more than what they see during clinic hours and who does not possess the depth of knowledge the patient's condition needs.

The most valuable move an NP or a PA can make for themselves or their career is put an honest effort into learning and mastering their craft. This step requires reading outside of clinic, looking up diagnostic entities when they are not sure of the treatment, and continual review of the literature. They must become a student of their craft.

Dedicating to a life of continual learning is imperative to being a quality provider. At the same time, it is essential to developing trust from the patient. The two sides of this thought process are that the knowledge is essential to being a quality provider, and that without the mastery and dedication, the patients know.

Thus, it is better to *be the person* you would want *to be seen by*. This philosophy should be sought out in new hires, (as indicated in an earlier chapter), reiterated in those who work with us, and should be exemplified by the supervising physician.

Take the opportunities to review new therapies, alternative approaches to diagnosis, or other items you read about with your NP or PA. The effort you put into sharing that you *too* read, study, and learn continually leaves no room for excuses from the other providers you mentor. Be the example.

It has been said a rising tide lifts all boats. Continually increase your own knowledge, and expect the same from your NP or PA. An unequivocal demand for knowledge and quality care will raise the level of the practice, because such dedication leads patients to trust you and your team. This is the step that lifts the tide for the medical office.

Chapter 24
Train a Limited-spectrum or Full-spectrum NP or PA?

There is a plethora of ways to train the NP or PA in dermatology. Planning is one of the key factors. As the supervising physician, you must determine what you want as the outcome.

If you are training for cosmetics, surgery, or medical dermatology, the path you choose might be different. For the sake of this book, we will focus on the medical dermatology, because that is what I have found is the core of most practices.

The amount of knowledge required to be proficient in medical dermatology is magnitudes more than learning only procedures. The medical component is not so much a skill, like injecting or suturing, but rather becoming a diagnostician, tactician, and implementer of plans. Not only does the medical dermatology provider have to be accurate in diagnosis, but he or she also must be able to change plans if the initial treatment regimen is not effective.

The providers who have extensive knowledgeable are often more confident and able to manage the nuances of the specialty.

So how exactly do we get them the knowledge? There are several ways, and the first order of business is determining which patients you want them to see.

Some dermatology practices follow "limited-spectrum" guidelines. They limit the NP or PA to seeing only acne, verrucae, and a few other conditions. This does not prove to be cost-effective in the long run, as patients invariably ask for other ailments to be looked at, diagnosed, and managed. Therefore, these types of practices will have the dermatologist see the patient and then have the follow-up scheduled with the NP or PA.

The opposite of the limited-spectrum practice guidelines is the practice that expects the NP or PA to practice like a dermatologist. In this "full-spectrum" situation, new patients, follow-ups, and urgent work-ins get put on the schedule of the NP or PA. This often allows the dermatologist to focus on other areas of expertise or preferred practice such as surgery, cosmetics, or more complicated dermatologic issues.

In the "full-spectrum" practice setting, the NP or PA must have enough knowledge to handle the failures of treatment on basic cases, know the differential well enough to recognize what is an expected norm versus a treatment failure, and have enough expertise to identify when to deploy further testing (i.e., biopsies, blood work, etc.).

Most dermatologists want the full-spectrum NP or PA. The hard part is that new hires with experience, solid knowledge in dermatology, and excellent practice methods are in high demand but short supply. Naturally, that leads to the dermatologist having to provide extensive training themselves.

This is not an easy process, but with a systematic approach it can be very rewarding for the dermatologist, the NP or PA, and the patient population.

Steps on how to train a new graduate are discussed in the upcoming chapters, based on experience not only in my own practice—where I have made it a mission to deploy only the highest quality providers for our patient population—but also the input of others.

My years of learning how to efficiently and effectively train NPs and PAs, and amassing data for that purpose, led me to create Dermwise to benefit fellow dermatologists. With testing in practices throughout the United States via our online Dermwise business, we have trained hundreds of medical providers who are new to the field, as well as dozens who have dermatology experience. As we developed and refined the program, it was run through alpha and beta testing, with feedback given from board-certified dermatologists and the participating NPs and PAs themselves. This group from around the country helped formulate additional ideas and concepts that have made training a dermatology NP or PA much more efficient.

In essence this book, combined with the Dermwise training, can do the heavy lifting, so to speak, allowing dermatologists to focus on patient care. However, if you prefer to shoulder training of your NP or PA yourself, the next several chapters will present valuable information used in Dermwise, so that you may be sure to cover all key bases.

If you would like more information about the online training program, visit www.dermwise.com.

Chapter 25
Competence
Creates Confidence

Public speaking has been rated as the greatest fear a person can have. Instructors of this craft quote studies that this fear is higher than even death. And yet, coaches and teachers in the realm of public speaking find a solution. How?

Well, if we understand some techniques of reducing this fear, we are in turn solving a problem that would otherwise hold people back.

Dale Carnegie wrote *How to Win Friends and Influence People* as well as *The Quick and Easy Way to Effective Public Speaking*. Part of his philosophy in overcoming the fear of public speaking was to talk only about a subject a person knows and understands very well. When the expert in the room on the topic is the person speaking, they can overcome many inhibitions and fears.

Being the expert in the room changes the dynamics from giving a speech into sharing a "talk." Giving a speech often reduces the engagement to a forced effort of memorizing canned words or reading from a transcript. The talk is a personal sharing of an individual's experience or knowledge, which they know better than anyone in the room. The results are often a message that is genuine and real.

Why is this relevant to training nurse practitioners and physician assistants? It is because providers must sit in the exam room with a patient, with or without family members or others present (in other words, an audience). The patient and their counterparts are looking for help and answers. The unfortunate truth for a new provider, as noted previously, is that the other people in the room can usually sniff out incompetence and ignorance quickly.

Thus, whether a physician, nurse practitioner, or physician assistant realizes it or not, a requisite for quality care includes *competence*.

There is no hiding incompetence or ignorance. The patient's mind cannot return to a time of not knowing. Acceptance is hard to come by when diagnosis or treatment regimens are inappropriate or wrongly recommended by a poorly trained person, in particular one who is trying to pass him- or herself off as a specialist.

To give a provider quality education is to give them competence. And yes, competence leads to confidence. Confidence then evokes trust in the patient, and this leads to a willingness to have a relationship for care.

A Competence Test

If you are wondering how many providers who walk into your office with primary care experience are likely to have actual dermatologic competence, consider this.

While writing this book, we interviewed several candidates for our office. One had interviewed two years ago and shared how passionate she was about dermatology, including investing in herself by learning about biopsy techniques at a nurse practitioner conference.

Another had been inspired to become a dermatology physician assistant two years ago. Because he was in the military, he was only given the option to do family practice, though he had asked about options for learning dermatology during his military training.

A third person wanted to pursue dermatology after spending three years as a nurse practitioner in the ICU and as a hospitalist. She indicated she had been inspired to do dermatology as a child when she spent time with her uncle, who was a dermatologist, and enjoyed reading his periodicals.

Each was given our Dermwise pretest of 100 questions, but not a single one scored higher than 55 percent. This is just three of the people we interviewed over the space of a year, all of whom expressed a passion for dermatology. Not a single one scored enough to be competent.

To put the scores into perspective, as of this writing the most recent ten participants who completed the Dermwise training averaged above a 95 percent on their post-test assessment.

This observation reminds us that wanting to be a dermatology provider and being a provider are different.

The late, great motivational speaker Zig Ziglar stated, "You've got to be before you can do, and do before you can have." In the medical world, physicians must go through so many steps that they are generally assumed to be competent. For NPs or PAs, the onus is on the physician to ensure that their providers are competent before they turn them loose them on their patients.

Having an objective, measurable method to validate knowledge is the best way to help NPs and PAs feel better about, and eventually have confidence in, their own abilities.

Therefore, it is important to create a system that helps the practice ensure each provider has competence in at least the academic realm of dermatology.

For those who do not wish to put in the time to build a system, the Dermwise training can be a consideration (yes, you may file this under "shameless plug"; I developed it so that no other physician would ever have to). To clarify, Dermwise was designed to provide the didactic component for NPs and PAs so physicians have significantly less of a burden in training their providers. Dermwise was also tailored to facilitate the dermatology provider having accountability for education.

Whether you use Dermwise or develop a system for yourself, make sure you 1) create a method that establishes an objective means of providing accountability. This can be done by creating a reading schedule, developing lectures with many visual images of not only the diagnosis but also the items in the differential diagnosis, and then creating tests to verify assimilation of topics taught. At the same time, 2) work to get your provider as competent, and thereby confident, as fast as you can.

The resulting competence will reveal itself as confidence that patients can believe in.

Chapter 26
Tailor Training to Achieve
Specific Outcomes

What is the type of provider/patient relationship you envision your NP or PA having? In other words, what type of patients or what type of diagnostic entities do you envision your NP or PA seeing, treating, and managing in your clinic?

Most dermatologists want to have their NP or PA see as many patients as possible, with as little involvement of the physician as is practical. In addition, most physicians want this to happen in just a few months.

Helping your provider attain the knowledge you feel is appropriate to begin seeing patients can occur via several paths. There is no "one way" to achieve your desired end result.

In some instances, physicians believe there should be a long narrow path, with no side roads or variations. An analogy might be when an adventurer takes to a trail on the side of a tall mountain where only the strongest can hike up. At the top, an old wise person is there to enlighten them. This enlightenment usually occurs after more work, time, and study have been completed. Thus, this trip took a great deal of time, and it culminated by reaching the summit. This scenario represents the physicians who believe an NP or a PA must have an incredible amount of knowledge before caring for patients.

There are other physicians who believe only a smidgen of knowledge is needed to cover the very basics of dermatology before they expect the provider to begin seeing patients. On the mountain of knowledge, they might jump off after the first mile marker, and then represent themselves as the same type of person who made their way to the top. Some physicians find a manner to utilize an NP or a PA with minimal dermatology proficiency.

The truth in medicine is that no nurse practitioner or physician assistant is going to have the training of a dermatologist. Their knowledge of the common can become quite strong if they put in effort and energy over many years, but it will not equal a dermatologist.

Physicians must determine the type of patients they are willing to allow their nurse practitioner or physician assistant to see. Some dermatologists control who sees their NP or PA by only having a certain type of established patients with specific diagnostic entities seen by them. Others will allow their providers to see any patient who comes in, which requires a broader spectrum of knowledge.

Determining the provider-patient relationship you want for your NP or PA is important. This will enable you to get a good idea of the outcome you want the training to achieve and the amount of training you want him or her to have.

Some physicians will train their NPs or PAs on a limited number of diagnostic entities, provide them a regimen of therapeutic options, and then screen the patients the NP or PA sees. Then the provider can be taught an algorithm to adjust therapy based on the response to the treatment rendered by the dermatologist. This allows the NP or PA to expand the number of patients being seen by the practice, even with a limited knowledge of dermatology. This occurs because the physician utilizes their own differential diagnostic skills to ensure an accurate diagnosis rather than depending on the NP or PA for this.

Situations where the dermatologist can assign the diagnosis and then transfer care via follow-up to the NP or PA might include entities such as acne, rosacea, atopic dermatitis, and psoriasis. The response to therapy can be evaluated at follow-up, and then the NP or PA can adjust the regimen based on a protocol devised by the dermatologist. Essentially the dermatologist is seeing the patient initially to properly diagnose, and then the follow-up is with the NP or PA.

The other spectrum of expectations occurs when the dermatologist expects the NP or PA to be capable of seeing each patient independently on the initial presentation to the office. In this scenario, the NP or PA must have the skills to formulate a differential diagnosis and then attain an accurate diagnosis. The NP or PA is thus functioning in a more autonomous manner.

It would seem obvious that a provider the dermatologist can trust to see patients independently is a more valuable addition to the practice. It is also one who requires more education, training, and supervision. This is the reason a well-trained, experienced provider is typically the goal of most dermatology physicians.

Most dermatology practices are thus looking to find or create the highly competent NP or PA in as little time as possible. It is not uncommon for practices to deploy a method of training that involves starting the NP or PA (who has limited experience) seeing patients who have known diagnostic entities that can be easily managed. As the provider gains knowledge and enhances the ability to formulate a differential diagnosis, they can manage a broader spectrum of entities.

The following chapters are going to outline techniques, tools, and study schedules that are designed to maximize the educational schedule goals for any NP or PA. The processes discussed will expedite the training process of your new NP or PA. In addition, the information can be just as valuable for enhancing the educational background of "experienced" providers. This is because many dermatology NPs or PAs practice dermatology, but often have not had nearly the dermatology education and training than one would expect.

The plan laid out for the education of a dermatology NP or PA going forward is designed to help provide a strong, solid fund of knowledge. This can help get an NP or a PA functioning on the basics in the shortest time possible. The fundamentals that are stressed in the following chapters can help providers build on their fund of knowledge and become more well-rounded at any stage of their training or career.

Chapter 27
Differential Diagnosis:
The Key to Mastering Dermatology

At times we may be tempted to think the NP or PA will be able to handle the patients who come into the office with ease. Of course, if that were the case, every primary care provider would hold on to their own acne, verrucae, rosacea, and skin cancer patients. Though that may be a desire, the truth is that a solid foundation of knowledge is needed to truly care for patients effectively. The fund of knowledge must be tied to something more.

What is the something more? It is the ability to categorize the findings the provider sees in the exam room and then formulate a differential diagnosis. Though this seems elementary to dermatologists, because most have made creating differentials second nature during their careers, this process is imperative for dermatology care. When training an NP or a PA, many dermatologists do not understand the importance of categorizing exam findings to facilitate differential diagnosis formation in day-to-day practice.

The ability to categorize lesions is crucial in teaching dermatology. It is the key when you want to have an NP or a PA who can treat the majority of your patients. It is a clear *must* that your provider learns how to formulate a differential diagnosis.

That sounds simple. We as dermatologists know it is not. In fact, the reason our post-medical school training is four years centers around knowing the zebra conditions.

Teaching a provider how to formulate a differential diagnosis, then, is a key to successful implementation of an NP or a PA.

The basic parameters of educating on this topic are much easier to understand if a system is put in place for them.

Building a system of differential diagnosis that helps a provider think like a dermatologist is quite possible. When we put on our teacher hats to educate our NPs or PAs, we must go back to teaching the very basics. This means for each topic or diagnostic entity, we must think of the scenario in which a mimic or lookalike could present. From there we need photographic images we can share with our NP or PA for each item in the differential diagnosis. Then we can teach why each of the items on the differential list is present.

This method of education enables a provider to become a diagnostician and tactician in the exam room. Becoming proficient in differential diagnosis formulation frees the provider up from making so many errors in diagnosis because they are intellectually engaged in identification.

Understanding differentials, though, requires educating in a broader manner than simply learning each diagnosis one at a time.

In order to learn differential diagnosis, the student must see the diagnosis they are being taught and the items in the differential. For example, a discussion of a papulosquamous condition, such as nummular dermatitis, should include other papulosquamous eruptions and the distinguishing factors morphologically and distributionwise (i.e., atopic dermatitis, psoriasis, guttate psoriasis, xerotic dermatitis, cutaneous lupus, and others). Then, as the education moves to other conditions in the same group, a review of the features of nummular dermatitis is brought up again.

Teaching in the differential diagnostic pattern would then allow for each time cutaneous lupus is brought up, a brief review of nummular dermatitis with photographic images is discussed. For each entity in the papulosquamous list, the other diagnostic conditions can thus be reviewed with photographic images.

This method of teaching yields several advantages. Seeing diagnostic entities multiple times helps through repetition. Seeing diagnostic entities in context of their categorization puts them in context, which causes engagement intellectually as part of the sorting process. Being shown the similarities and differences in the primary lesions, morphology, and distribution leaves a more lasting impression.

Education focused on differential diagnosis formation gives a faster method of learning, a more solid base from which to grow, and lays a foundation the supervising physician can trust.

In my own personal experience of training NP and PA students, medical students, and rotating primary care residents, this method has been by far the best approach to turning the light on. Over years of generating content for the Indiana University Medical Students as Dermatology Clerkship Director, I have heard medical students who are taught through the categorization (differential diagnostic) method rave about how they understand so much more of dermatology than before. This method works, and it is the cornerstone for the building of quality NP and PA providers in dermatology.

Over time and through multiple teaching opportunities, the method of categorization (differential diagnostic) instruction has become a cornerstone for my mode of training. As my dermatology colleagues learned of this training system, they began asking me to share it with their NP or PAs. This is what led to the development of the online training system at Dermwise. The Dermwise training—absolutely shameless plug, because the training is so effective—emphasizes the differential diagnosis for each entity through many photographic images, discussion of the rationale for each diagnosis, and clues to correct diagnosis. The categorization (differential diagnosis) process is emphasized with every single topic and module in the training.

After being educated on the differential as the basis for learning, the provider can then start thinking of a differential when entering the exam room. The categorization method is thus the most important foundational concept for any dermatology provider. The benefit for the supervising physician who has a provider trained in this modality is that the NP or PA is grown into a true dermatology provider.

Chapter 28
Differential Diagnosis:
Teach Upside-down Medical Care

"I would give a discount if the patient did not talk," quipped a satirical comment from a dermatology instructor who was trying to make a point during my residency training. For fear it might embarrass him, I will not reveal who it was, but I can say he was one of those fellows who has written several books and is renowned.

His comment came when he was teaching us the basis of formulating a differential diagnosis. It was said to make a point and draw a laugh from dermatology residents who felt they were overworked and exhausted from learning. The reality of his comment has stood out to me over time, though, because of the follow-up he shared with us.

He reminded us that without a patient saying a word, the differential diagnosis should be formulated. This was upside down from what all of the other medical professionals had trained us to do, over and over, for the last four years of medical school and one year of internship. Only after going through the three years of dermatology training did the reason for his comment come to light, as it has for almost every dermatologist.

The time to do the physical exam is when we walk in the room, though patients would feel that is awkward. So, we exchange pleasantries and talk briefly about history while we try to get a peek at why they are coming to see us. After we see what the primary lesion is, we then formulate a differential diagnosis.

It is after the differential diagnosis is formulated that the *real* history can be elicited.

It is the pattern seen by almost every dermatology professional's office in the country. It is not the pattern any non-dermatologist provider is ever trained to do.

It becomes part of our responsibility to enlighten the NP or PA we have hired to start thinking accurately. As Zig Ziglar once said, "There is no room for stinking thinkin'." It is up to us to train our provider how to accurately assess patients and then properly manage their care.

Whether we hire an NP or a PA who has experience or is just beginning their dermatology career, we must teach them what some would view as upside-down medical care. They must learn to quickly identify the primary lesion through evaluation of cutaneous findings (using the eyes), then formulate a differential (learned via categorization methods), and finally determine the diagnosis (picking the right item from the differential). This process occurs when a dermatology provider is thinking accurately. And accurate thinking leads to the correct diagnosis.

Take the time to teach your provider categorization (differential diagnosis formulation), and your patients, and thus your practice, will benefit from a properly trained provider.

Chapter 29
Differential Diagnosis:
Full Skin Exam—Fact or Myth?

A key for providers who are new to the world of dermatology is to understand the value of a full-cutaneous skin exam.

Some dermatologists and most primary care providers will allow patients to remain fully clothed during the office visit. This can be a horrendous mistake for the provider who has limited training. Discerning psoriasis from seborrheic dermatitis might very well be a limited factor for the patient presenting with a scalp rash, since your treatment will likely be quite similar for both. But the patient who presents with a rash on the face who also has annular and oval plaques on the chest and back might be misdiagnosed with rosacea when they actually have lupus. Or the patient who presents with a rash on the hands but the feet are not evaluated can be misdiagnosed with a hand eczema when they have dermatophytosis.

At times, the distribution of lesions is key in finding the accurate diagnosis. The best method to observe distribution is to train the NP or PA to do full examinations on as many patients as possible. The full exam might not find anything that helps, but it trains the NP or PA to be thorough, consider a wider range in the differential, and not focus to quickly on one diagnosis.

Like most dermatologists, I have found a plethora of skin cancers on sites that are covered by clothes when the patient walks in the room complaining about the benign seborrheic keratosis on the hand or forehead. It is only through my compulsion to have our medical team request patients put on a gown for a full skin examination that we have found many of these cancers.

One example used in my teaching slides is of a man in his sixties who came in for telangiectasias of the nose. He initially resisted a full exam but was found to have a melanoma on the upper back when he allowed me to examine him.

As mentors and trainers of NPs and PAs, part of making sure patients get quality care is performing full cutaneous examinations. This identifies more skin cancers than we might imagine and thus can save lives. At the same time, this practice helps the NP or PA continually think in terms of differential diagnosis and distribution when evaluating the patient.

The utilization of full cutaneous skin examinations also highlight the understanding of lesion distribution. So far, we have discussed essentially primary lesions and presentations of patients for categorization and differential diagnosis formation. A thorough examination on every patient possible can begin to solidify the component of distribution for your NP or PA.

In the learning phase, your NP or PA needs to see the varied locations and presentations of diseases so they begin to appreciate the classic presentations as well as the variants of common disease entities. When a patient presents with psoriasis and has classic silvery scaled plaques on the elbows and knees, but also has moist non-scaling plaques in the inframammary area consistent with inverse psoriasis, the provider would only see the intertriginous presentation if doing a full exam.

After seeing lesions of psoriasis under the breast multiple times, the provider should be able to formulate a differential diagnosis for pink plaques. At the same time, understanding distribution means they should look at the scalp so they can determine if the patient has psoriasis. In the patient who presents concerned about inframammary confluent pink plaques, the provider would know to consider not only intertrigo, but also inverse psoriasis. They might find that one of the beauties of performing a full exam is being able to utilize distribution of lesions as an adjuvant agent in diagnosis.

In the book *Accelerated Learning* by Colin Rose, the process of organization, restructuring, and placement of learned tasks into groups was found to be a powerful method of learning. With the amount of knowledge a new provider is expected to assimilate, utilizing scientifically proven methods of rapid learning is vital. Taking advantage of these techniques is the core of what we are discussing here.

In your training of the NP or PA, it is imperative to teach categorization (differential diagnosis formation) and distribution at the beginning of training. When taught at the beginning, these items become foundational cornerstones from which you can build. Combining the efficiencies of science-based learning with practical dermatology can escalate and accelerate the abilities of your NP or PA.

Chapter 30
Education Planning:
Pick the Book and Start with Basics

For almost every medical specialty, there is a gold standard for the textbook that a purist should learn from, in order to be considered proficient. Because these textbooks are full of detail, minutia, and facts, they initially overwhelm resident physicians, even after four years of medical school. First-year residents in dermatology have a difficult time assimilating and learning *Fitzpatrick's Dermatology in General Medicine*, in part because of the depth in which each topic is covered. It is challenging to learn all the fine details without first having a general overview of the topics.

Perhaps the powers that be in the realm of academia have discerned this. Some larger textbooks are now being distributed in a more manageable format, such as *Dermatology* by Bolognia. Even though some say Bolognia's text flows more smoothly and is an easier read than many other resource textbooks, the fact that it is quite large makes it a challenge to use as an introduction to the specialty.

In understanding the challenges residents (even ourselves, in the first year of residency) face, we must take a step back and look at which book might be best for a physician assistant or nurse practitioner to learn our specialty. As we consider possibilities, we must recognize the mentality and training differences between NP/PAs and medical doctors.

Physicians have worked seven-day weeks with days of twelve to twenty-four hours of patient care and responsibility.

This time commitment is not required of any other professionals in medicine. So, during their education process, an NP or a PA has not been required to spend the same time studying that a physician might have dedicated. This is not a detriment, but rather a fact that supervising physicians must recognize.

Thus, it is important to look back at your own training, think about which text items were most helpful, and see if one is appropriate for an NP or a PA. Ideally, the book would have a solid overview, provide guides as a reference, be rapidly consumed, and act as a comprehensive tool of education. The book should be acceptable for someone who has minimal to no knowledge of dermatology but can provide a solid foundation for the basics of dermatology.

One of the most popular books for this, in my experience, is *Andrews' Diseases of the Skin: Clinical Dermatology*. Though it does not have as much detail as the so-called reference books, it is a resource that provides a good, basic understanding of dermatology.

Some dermatologists want to use one of the larger, thick reference text books as the study guide. Again, one must remember that the content must be manageable and digestible in a rapid amount of time.

The Andrew's book provides what we are looking for, in a 10,000-foot view, or a look from the treetops, so to speak. Therefore, we are providing the basics as our first order of business.

In the Dermwise training system, a methodology termed "Tree Learning" is taught. With this, we use the tree as an analogy. The roots and trunk of a tree must be healthy and strong in order for the branches and leaves to be vibrant and healthy. In learning a new specialty, there are basics that must be mastered, and the basics provide the roots and trunk, or core of knowledge. It is with this core that the new items can be grown from.

The so-called branches and leaves are the specifics, which at times can be overwhelming. The fine details, esoteric facts, and layers of knowledge physicians have pushed into their minds are difficult to attain and maintain until a foundation is laid from which to build. As the process of learning unfolds, the roots grow deeper and stronger.

Viewing learning in this manner is similar to how nature protects and grows the strongest trees. A powerful root system and solid trunk help support so much more as time progresses.

Placing our educational system on a foundation of basics can help our providers have more confidence and resources to pull from, just like the tree with strong roots and trunk can withstand high winds or torrential downpours of strong storms.

Too many providers and physicians think the minute details, aka leaves in our tree analogy, are the place to start teaching. Unfortunately this leads to a future without a firm understanding of the core principles. This in turn can cause more errors in diagnosis, can result in patient care errors, and in the end can potentially leave both the supervising physician and the NP or PA in line of potential legal consequences.

It is best, then, to find the right resources and invest some time to provide basics of knowledge. Medical competency starts with fundamental mastery.

There are many resources and options to train an NP or a PA. A combination of one or several textbooks is often necessary to be used for lectures, discussion, and reference. There is no one text that encompasses all of what any provider must master, but there are some that I have found helpful, and in discussion with other dermatologists have found agreement.

The Andrew's book heads the list as a study guide and text for the NP or PA. Our providers are given the latest and most up-to-date copy of *Andrews' Diseases of the Skin: Clinical Dermatology* upon their hire. The required reading for them is from this text, and the chapters are not too overwhelming for a beginner. It provides a manageable amount of information, which is excellent for the NP or PA to use as a base textbook.

At the same time, we have found *Dermatology* by Bolognia, and *Comprehensive Dermatologic Drug Therapy* textbooks are extremely useful for assigned reading as well as resource textbooks.

Another point to consider is some textbooks, including the *Andrews' Diseases of the Skin: Clinical Dermatology, Dermatology* (by Bolognia), and *Comprehensive Dermatologic Drug Therapy* textbooks, may be purchased as a print or e-book version with additional online availability. This has been useful for our providers as we have computers throughout the office including examination rooms. When a question arises, such as alternative therapies to granuloma annulare, the provider may log in to the online textbook and have access to the textbook.

To help facilitate finding images for teaching differential diagnosis, one can consider online searches/sites, color atlases of dermatology, and a resource available in an online and text format termed *VisualDx*. These tools can help provide images to teach the skills of differential diagnosis formulation.

Another educational tool our providers have found helpful, in particular during the early phases of training, includes the differential diagnosis card stack *Dermatology DDX Deck*. It is a printed rack of cards that is longitudinal and narrow, and fastened at one end so that different cards can be fanned out and looked at simultaneously. Each card has a few pictures of a diagnosis listed on it and a brief synopsis of the condition. This tool helps solidify the categorization method of thinking.

As you can imagine, there are many textbooks, resources, and tools that can be used to educate your NP or PA. One of the chief factors is finding something that ensures the time you, as an instructor, utilize is most efficient. Simultaneously, the method of education must be concise, powerful, and grow your provider rapidly.

The items I specify in this chapter are the tools I have found most helpful. If you are more familiar with different resources or texts, one may be better for you. The aim in picking resources for training the NP or PA is to maximize the dermatologist's time, the student/trainee's time, and achieve the end result of great quality care.

A list of some of the resources I have found helpful includes those on the next page.

Teaching Resources, in Order of My Personal Preference

- *Andrews' Diseases of the Skin: Clinical Dermatology.* William D. James, MD, Timothy Berger, MD, Dirk Elston, MD.
- *Dermatology.* Jean L. Bolognia, MD, Joseph L. Jorizzo, MD, Julie V. Schaffer, MD.
- *Comprehensive Dermatologic Drug Therapy.* Stephen E. Wolverton.
- *Dermatology DDx Deck.* Thomas P. Habif, MD, James L. Campbell, Jr., MD.
- *Clinical Dermatology: A Color Guide to Diagnosis and Therapy.* Thomas P. Habif, MD.
- *Dermatology Essentials.* Jean L. Bolognia, MD, Julie V. Schaffer, MD, Karynne O. Duncan, MD, Christine J. Ko, MD.
- *Fitzpatrick's Dermatology in General Medicine.* Lowell A. Goldsmith, MD, Klaus Wolff, MD, and others.
- *VisualDx: Essential Adult Dermatology (VisualDx: The Modern Library of Visual Medicine).* Lowell A. Goldsmith, MD, Art Papier, MD.

Chapter 31
Practice, Trust, and Verify

It is important to pair the discussion of educational resources with a brief synopsis of making good use of them—in other words, practice, trust, and verify.

As you can imagine, the first few months of an NP or a PA's hire is a bit overwhelming for them. When they seem to reach the point of getting their wits about them and gaining some knowledge of dermatology, we must remember some strategies to keep them growing.

Science is often about proving theories right and wrong. In medicine, providers must learn to become scientists who search for answers and look up information themselves. This is a core factor in becoming a competent provider, since medicine is a lifetime of learning. For this reason, supervising physicians must encourage, and even demand, our NPs and PAs self-educate.

If you feel a new hire can be trusted with your patients, you are probably right. There are so many NPs and PAs who are competent, hard-working, and willing to pay the price to be a great provider that you will be pleased to have made the choice of hiring them.

At the same time, it is important to have the new hire practice what they are doing, continually study what they have seen, and improve their knowledge daily. As with most humans, the best scenario is to have a mentor support and also push the provider.

In our clinic, this means the supervising physician should ask questions of the NP or PA after seeing a challenging case, then follow up the next day. The questions should center around something important for a good dermatology provider to be aware of, such as asking what laboratory monitoring is required of someone taking dapsone, or inquiring what are the side effects of being on minocycline for prolonged periods of time.

The follow-up the next day is vital to learning. It makes the NP or PA know that someone is counting on them to look up the data about the diagnosis or treatment plan. If the supervising physician can make this a consistent process, the NP or PA gets into the habit of researching what they do not know or have an answer for. The importance of the physician follow-up cannot be underscored enough.

Eventually a pattern of behavior develops that is, at the very core, education-oriented. This method of case-based learning is so powerful that some medical schools are even moving toward a systematic process requiring integration of didactic and clinical scenarios. This method teaches your NP or PA to be resourceful in looking up the challenges of their own patients or areas of concern. After consistently proving to the physician that the behavior is one of continued self-education, trust can be built between the supervising physician and the provider.

The trust of a physician knowing his NP or PA is studying conditions and cases of the day is reassuring to both parties. It is also a cornerstone of quality care.

Just like any habit, though, learning in a continual manner requires verification. The supervising physician should make it a point to continually ask questions, follow up on the inquiries, and expect excellence. The standard of care should be high, and demands for such are not unreasonable. The process of practice, verify, and trust are thus important for the physician and NP or PA relationship.

On a separate level, for the NP or PA who is working more independently, this process is essential for themselves. The highest level of care is achieved when the NP or PA is working diligently on their knowledge, and thus the practice. At the same time, it is best when they are utilizing the available resource textbooks in a verification process. This leads to a situation where the patient is placed in the hands of someone they can trust. In the end, the practicing and verifying of patient care will lead to exemplary care from every provider.

Chapter 32
A Sample Week of Training

If you are hiring a new graduate, someone who has been practicing in another specialty, or someone whose experience you want to verify, expect a minimum of two to three months before they can typically add value to your clinic.

Textbook Assignments

To begin instructing your provider, take your textbook of choice and jot down the chapters you feel are the absolute essentials to caring for your patients. Now, as a dermatologist, there may not be any chapters you would view as second tier, but in training the NP or PA, you must prioritize the process.

The art of dermatology requires understanding the basics of physiology, skin anatomy, and dermatologic terminology. From there one must learn the art of categorizing lesions.

Pick the chapters that you feel are the type of diagnostic entities your provider will start off seeing.

Ideally, if you hire your NP or PA two to three months before they are to start work in your office, you can assign the provider the list of general topics to read and prepare for before they arrive at your clinic (getting them past the basics). This would allow them to begin education on specific topics at the time of arrival.

Upon arrival, to make the process go as smoothly as possible, a pattern we have found helpful is to assign one chapter/topic per week from a dermatology textbook. (This works quite well with *Andrews' Diseases of the Skin: Clinical*

Dermatology.) The requirement is not simply to read, but to study and master the content.

Once the provider has the basics and has learned and mastered the fundamentals, specific diagnostic entities or more specific chapters can be brought forward as topics to learn and master.

Exams Based on the Textbook Material

At the end of the week, have the NP/PA take an exam over the content. An exam helps verify the content is mastered, not simply read. An exam also helps motivate the NP or PA to remain diligent in their studies.

The value of examinations cannot be underscored enough. If the NP or PA isn't held accountable to learning, the provider may be dead weight in the office until they do.

And when an NP or a PA consistently struggles with attaining the proficiency necessary, we must consider the cost of keeping them on board. Obviously, paychecks are given out to the provider, but also your time investment, the loss of patients, the practice reputation, and staff investment in time helping acclimate the new provider to the office are all impacted when the provider fails to effectively gain knowledge in the specialty.

Weekly Meeting

Immediately following the exam each week, a mandatory one-on-one meeting between the physician and NP/PA should take place, each thirty to sixty minutes in length.

The ideal scenario is to make each educational session as high yield for the new hire as possible and the least burdensome for the dermatologist. It is best for the physician to read the chapter though beforehand.

For the duration of the time slot, both you and the NP or PA must be focused on the educational process and must minimize digressions.

During each meeting, it is important to review the important points from the previous week's assigned educational material and discuss any difficulties as indicated by the exam. For the dermatologist, the clinical aspects that are utilized day in and day out in regard to the topic can provide added content for the educational session.

If there are scripts you tell your patients about a given topic, these can be briefly shared during the meetings, but the medical assistants and nurses who routinely disseminate this information can also help share it with the new NP or PA. Then you can simply describe the "why" in your sessions and verify that the NP/PA has gained the knowledge required.

An example might be explaining how to apply topical retinoids. In our practice, we encourage washing the face, waiting thirty to sixty minutes, and then applying one green pea size of tretinoin (or other retinoid) for the entire face. A new hire can hear me say this to patients, and then hear it reiterated by the medical assistants. They can take in what the medical assistants have learned, and then have the dermatologist discuss the rationale. Learning the "why" is imperative for the NP or PA.

Sample Session

The following sample session uses a thirty-minute learning time. Each session, whether thirty or sixty minutes, can be broken down into thirds. (Again, the follow session can be prefaced with a review of the previous week's assigned material and any issues the week's exam revealed. What follows is strictly time for learning new material.)

First 10 minutes: It should be relatively easy for you to give a ten-minute synopsis. For example, if the topic is acne, you can review the ages of onset, basic etiology, types of lesions, and your typical treatment algorithm based on types of lesions/presentations.

Second 10 minutes: Ask if there are any questions. Review any components the provider has questions about or needs clarification on.

Third 10 minutes: Ask fixed questions. These can be open-ended and provide opportunities for discussion. The remaining minutes can then use utilized to go through the next chapter in the textbook, with you directing discussion on the topics you feel to be most relevant.

Again, this thirty minutes would need to be highly efficient and focused entirely on education. Clearly it is not enough to get a provider up and going in short order, but it can be an intense, high-yield session if done properly, resulting in effective learning.

We, along with other physicians we have spoken to, believe a minimum of one, if not more, of these meetings should occur each week. As you can imagine, doing this twice per week, or at least sixty minutes per week, can be even more impactful for the NP or PA.

Chapter 33
A Sample Schedule of
Weekly Training

We have tried varied methods of training, and honed in on the pattern that we have consistently seen produces the highest yield.

The training schedule includes one main chapter and module per week. The anchor is the Dermwise training system, which has corresponding assignments for reading in *Andrews' Diseases of the Skin: Clinical Dermatology* as the text. We also keep Bolognia's *Dermatology* text available. As previously noted, both can be purchased with online access availability.

A synopsis of our weekly training is outlined below.

Weekly Training

Monday: The educational assignment involves the weekly Dermwise Online Training video module, which the NP or PA is responsible for completing. Each video module is 1 to 1.5 hours and has corresponding textbook assignments in *Andrews' Diseases of the Skin: Clinical Dermatology* by James or *Dermatology* by Bolognia. The NP or PA is thus required to complete the video module and reading of the chapter. These activities do not require the presence of the dermatologist.

Wednesday Physician-Provider Session: The supervising physician meets with the NP or PA about midweek to go over a differential diagnosis (DDx) session. During this session, the physician shares images of the entities covered in the Dermwise module and assigned reading for the week. Initially, the focus is on building the dermatology vocabulary. As knowledge grows, the diagnostic entities become more of the focus. With continued progression, the ability to formulate a differential diagnosis occurs.

Thursday: The NP or PA takes the Dermwise exam, which corresponds to the module and assigned reading for the week.

Friday Physician-Provider Session: The supervising physician and provider review the week of learning, including practical tips and pointers from material learned in the chapter. They also review weak points from the exam, if any are identified. This is a time to share clinical pearls and touch on important points from the learning assignments.

This didactic process is a highly intense educational endeavor for an NP or a PA. The provider must be focused, dedicated, and committed to take on the level of learning.

The supervising physician who uses the Dermwise training system does not have to prepare lectures and exams, as these are part of the system. The dermatologist is responsible for the DDx session, which I personally keep to 30 minutes on Wednesdays, and another 30- to 60-minute session on Fridays to review the weekly learning.

Corresponding Clinical Process

From a clinical perspective, the NP or PA learns the office dynamics and software the first few weeks. Then he or she is given several new patients to see, present to me, and afterward we go in together and the visit occurs. For billing purposes, all history is taken again by myself and a full examination is performed again. All billing requirements are met to bill the patient under the physician.

The NP or PA is gradually given more patients and more responsibility.

This process is designed to acclimate them to the office, software, staff, and at the same time coincide with a rapid escalation of dermatology knowledge (in tandem with the educational schedule).

Sample Week

Activities each day of the week:

Daily	NP or PA in clinic seeing patients
	• follows me as shadow *or* sees own patients and presents them to me
	• as much patient contact time as possible
Daily	Charting review
	• teach documentation of lesion type and how to place dermatology notes in the chart
	▫ as provider knowledge grows, this requires less physician involvement
	• physician review and recommendation of changes/updates on charting
Daily	Review of any patient questions
	• ideally, teach points that correspond to Dermwise Training Module and assigned reading to maximize retention of weekly assignments

Recurring activities each week:

Monday	Dermwise Quick Start Online Dermatology Training module videos (1 to 1.5 hours) • NP or PA does online, on his or her own • NP or PA reads assigned chapter from *Andrews' Diseases of the Skin: Clinical Dermatology*
Wednesday	Physician-Provider Differential Diagnosis Session (Derm DDx) • review images of entities corresponding to Dermwise module and assigned reading • 30-minute session
Thursday	Dermwise exam • NP or PA takes an online exam for the assigned module and assigned reading
Friday	Physician-Provider Review Session • Physician and NP or PA review relevant points corresponding to Dermwise module and assigned reading

Chapter 34
Twelve-week High-intensity Training

Creating an educational schedule is key in laying out expectations for the NP or PA and in providing a structure to the training process. We have found utilizing a twelve-week system is best. This is because most professionals have had twelve-week semesters in school and accept the expectation of a high level of intensity for this duration.

Secondly, this tandems the ninety-day window that most businesses have as a probationary status. This allows the practice to determine if the new hire is making sufficient progress in the first ninety days.

In our practice, we coordinate the textbook chapters with online video modules from Dermwise. (The premise of the Dermwise training is to provide the most rapid foundation of knowledge for a new NP or PA. It is also useful for most experienced NP or PAs, because very few are taught proper differential diagnosis methodology and algorithmic approaches to cutaneous findings.)

The twelve-week cycle we have found most useful is as follows.

Week 1: Skin Basic Structure and Function—Disease processes are related to skin anatomy and cutaneous response. Image evaluation and explanation of thickening of the skin in callus formation and prurigo. Topical steroid utilization in relation to potency and side effects when used on the volar skin in contrast to eyelids. Embryologic development of the skin in relation to inherited conditions such as ichthyosis vulgaris and keratosis pilaris. Basal cell carcinoma formation in relation to basal cell biology in the epidermis. Melanocyte formation, biology, anatomy, and relation to nevi, melanoma, and vitiligo. Allergic contact dermatitis and urticaria biology, including relation to urticaria. A variety of other dermatologic conditions are touched on with description and photographic images, offering a broad overview of multiple conditions and how each relates to the anatomy and physiology of the skin.

Reading:

- *Andrews' Diseases of the Skin: Clinical Dermatology*— Skin Basic Structure and Function.
- And/or Bolognia's *Dermatology*—Section: Overview of Basic Science.

As you can see, the basic science of the skin can be used to provide an introduction to a multitude of cutaneous diseases. Building a familiarity and then a foundation of the common diseases is key in gaining strong clinical skills rapidly. If you elect to do this yourself, it is best to find images of clinical conditions that you can relate to the anatomy and physiology of the skin. Providing a clinical correlation to the basic science can help facilitate a strong foundation to build on going forward.

Week 2: Communicating in Dermatology—The process of learning the language of dermatology requires knowing extremely well how to describe cutaneous findings. It is imperative providers know and use proper descriptions. This occurs through knowing primary and secondary lesions.

To learn the primary and secondary lesions, providers should be familiar with the definitions, how terms are related, and common diagnostic entities. To make the knowledge more memorable, the techniques as described in the book *Accelerated Learning* by Colin Rose can be employed.

Memory-retention techniques include the techniques of repetition, organization, visual imagery, relationship building, and connecting to knowledge already attained. For this topic, it means studying many examples of images and reviewing why each lesion is in the primary or secondary category.

Review and repetition of many conditions with primary and secondary lesions, in addition to their relationship to each other descriptively, can improve retention. The key to the process is images, understanding, and relating items together.

Diagnostic entities and their relationship examples can include things such as defining a papule while sharing images of:

- congenital nevus
- dermal nevus
- cherry angioma
- molluscum contagiosum
- follicular eczema

The NP/PA should be able to define the entities with papules as well as describe some of the etiology, clinical features, and treatment. This process can help the student become familiar with not only communicating terminology but also with diagnostic conditions.

Follow papules with plaques, including examples of entities such as:

- congenital nevus
- seborrheic keratosis
- irritated seborrheic keratosis
- basal cell carcinoma
- psoriasis
- urticaria

Then, sharing the relationship and definition of a papule to a plaque reinforces the usage of dermatology terminology.

The key to this method of teaching is to find many examples, reiterate them frequently, and share information about the condition or diagnosis at each mention. This repetition increases familiarity and enhances speed of knowledge acquisition. The more quickly the NP or PA attains a base of knowledge, the more quickly they will become an asset in the clinic.

Reading:

- *Andrews' Diseases of the Skin, Clinical Dermatology*—Cutaneous Signs and Diagnosis.
- *Dermatology*—Section: Basic Principles of Dermatology.

Week 3: Power Categories to Correct Diagnosis—After mastering primary and secondary lesions, an NP or a PA must be able to categorize lesions. This is essential in the process of formulating a differential diagnosis. Though this seems straightforward to a dermatologist, the concept must be drilled repetitively for beginners to master it.

Creating the habit of identifying primary lesions, defining them, and utilizing this information to formulate a differential diagnosis is the core of accurate dermatology diagnosis. Finding a way to stimulate a new NP or PA to think in this manner—with each patient encountered—is critical. For this reason we, as supervising physicians, must structure training at every turn to come back to this principle.

The categorization process is essentially one of the core fundamentals of practicing dermatology. For the person who plays sports, be it golf, tennis, or basketball, to the person who plays a musical instrument, there are core fundamentals that must be mastered and practiced repeatedly for maximum performance. It is imperative we as dermatologists reinforce the usage of fundamentals frequently.

In the Dermwise program, the diseases are placed into what are termed Power Categories, which act as a foundational principle. The basis is essentially teaching the NP or PA to think morphologically and then place entities into appropriate categories.

Examples of the categories include:

- brown macules
- brown papules
- brown plaques
- red papules
- white macules
- gyrate and configurate lesions
- papulosquamous lesions

Knowledge of the categories provides a skeleton or structure for the NP or PA. The categories give a relational basis for all new entities as they are learned.

Repetition is key! For this reason, Week 3 is one in which lists of diagnostic entities can be categorized. Images of these entities can be reviewed, and then showing images of each item in the differential can be performed.

This provides multiple images, shows different aspects of lesions/conditions, and familiarizes the student with multiple diagnostic entities though broad exposure.

This familiarizes and reinforces the student so that more in-depth knowledge can be attained.

Reading:

- *Andrews' Diseases of the Skin, Clinical Dermatology*—Cutaneous Signs and Diagnosis.
- *Dermatology*—Section: Clinical and Pathological Differential.

Week 4: Pruritus and Neurodermatitis—The conditions that are described as having pruritus are many. This week is used to teach the basic science of pruritus and the conditions that are associated. At the same time, each entity should be coordinated with images and discussion of each of the items in the differential diagnosis.

Reading:
- *Andrews' Diseases of the Skin, Clinical Dermatology*—Pruritus and Neurocutaneous Dermatosis.
- *Dermatology*—Section: Pruritus.

Week 5: Atopic Dermatitis and Eczema—The topics discussed this week are crucial in terms of understanding etiology, course, and therapy. The Power Categories discussion for differential diagnosis during this week lends well to the conversation of distribution for disease diagnosis.

Beginners and experienced providers both absolutely must learn the papulosquamous entities. Atopic dermatitis is a cornerstone diagnosis for this category. Providers need to master the morphology, distribution, and variants of the diverse forms of eczema. At the same time, it is essential they learn the entities in the differential diagnosis.

The manner in which the information is presented for this week is crucial in laying a foundation for growth and understanding. Be sure to teach the papulosquamous conditions in the differential, in order to establish a platform from which to build knowledge going forward.

Reading:
- *Andrews' Diseases of the Skin, Clinical Dermatology*—Atopic Dermatitis and Eczema.
- *Dermatology*—Section: Atopic Dermatitis and Other Eczematous Eruptions.

Week 6: Urticaria, Angioedema, and Erythema—The basis for this week is learning the clinical presentation of urticaria, including proper diagnosis and therapy. If the NP or PA has been in another field, the predisposition to using prednisone as a basis for treatment is likely present. In this instance, "unteaching" may be necessary.

In addition, the topics of angioedema, erythema multiforme, drug eruption, and toxic epidermal necrolysis are important to grasp. These topics are part of this week's reading assignment.

Figurate erythemas can be a critical differential diagnosis category to review since urticaria is part of the differential. The fact that some of the gyrate and configurate erythema conditions scale, and others do not, can be a critical concept to understand.

This section is a wonderful time to educate about erythema without scale, in addition to the gyrate and configurate erythemas, with and without scale.

Reading:

- *Andrews' Diseases of the Skin, Clinical Dermatology*— Erythema and Urticaria.
- *Dermatology*—Sections: Urticaria and Angioedema. Figurate Erythemas. Erythema Multiforme and Toxic Epidermal Necrolysis. Eosinophilic Disorders and Neutrophilic Disorders.

Week 7: Seborrheic Dermatitis and Psoriasis—These two conditions, which serve as backbones of understanding much of dermatology, are critical to gain proficiency in, due to the high number of patients in whom these conditions appear in the differential diagnosis.

The diagnostic entities in these chapters of the textbook are significant, and attaining familiarity with the uncommon as well as mastering the common is imperative. Among other basics, it provides the opportunity to teach distribution of lesions, and type of scale (thick silvery/white for psoriasis versus the yellow greasy scale of seborrheic dermatitis). And again, this is an opportune week to educate regarding the differential diagnosis of papulosquamous entities.

Reading:

- *Andrews' Diseases of the Skin, Clinical Dermatology*— Seborrheic Dermatitis. Psoriasis. Recalcitrant Palmoplantar Eruptions. Pustular Dermatitis. Erythroderma.
- *Dermatology*—Section: Psoriasis and Other Papulosquamous Disorders.

Week 8: Pityriasis Rosea and the Other P's—The diagnosis of pityriasis rosea can seem straight forward to an experienced provider, but describing and showing the typical lesion morphology and distribution is important to the new provider.

Understanding the primary lesion, type of scale, and papulosquamous differential diagnosis is imperative, and this section provides the opportunity to again to review the entities within the differential diagnosis.

Topics covered in the reading also include pityriasis alba, parapsoriasis, pityriasis lichenoides chronica, and pityriasis lichenoides et varioliformis acuta, among others.

Reading:

- *Andrews' Diseases of the Skin, Clinical Dermatology*— Pityriasis Rosea, Pityriasis Rubra Pilaris, and Other Papulosquamous and Hyperkeratotic Diseases.
- *Dermatology*—Section: Other Papulosquamous Disorders.

Week 9: Lichen Planus and Related Conditions—As has been noted with many of the topics so far, the papulosquamous differential is reviewed again here. If it has not already been reviewed, the different types of scale—such as lichenoid, psoriasiform, and furfuraceous—can be reviewed and discussed. In addition, medication induction of lesions for lichen planus should be discussed.

Though one might think the diagnosis is direct, the condition yields itself well to discussion of medication induction of rashes, oral pathology (from Wickham's striae to ulcers/erosions and diseases that cause this), and nail changes.

Other conditions in the reading for this week include erythema dyschromicum perstans, lichen nitidus, lichen striatus, lichen sclerosus et atrophicus, and lichen planopilaris. The differential for each of these entities also leads to a broader discussion of possibilities.

Reading:
- *Andrews' Diseases of the Skin, Clinical Dermatology*— Lichen Planus and Related Conditions.
- *Dermatology*—Sections: Lichen Planus and Lichenoid Dermatosis. Pigmentary Disorders. Alopecia.

Week 10: Acne, Rosacea, and Variants—Acne, rosacea, and perioral dermatitis are such staples of the dermatology practice that this section may be one of the most important for an NP or a PA. The components of discussion can vary from diagnosis, differential diagnosis, and therapy to side effects of therapy, aggravating factors, and medication monitoring (such as for isotretinoin).

Some of the other entities discussed can include acne keloidalis, gram negative folliculitis, acne excoriée, hidradenitis suppurativa, dissecting cellulitis of the scalp, steroid dermatitis, and more.

Reading:

- *Andrews' Diseases of the Skin, Clinical Dermatology*— Acne.
- *Dermatology*—Sections: Acne Vulgaris. Rosacea and Related Conditions. Folliculitis and Other Follicular Disorders.

Week 11: Actinic Keratosis and Nonmelanoma Skin Cancer—It goes almost without saying that a provider of dermatology must be proficient at accurate diagnosis and treatment of actinic keratosis, basal cell carcinoma, and squamous cell carcinoma. The differential for each item is worth reviewing, including discussion of clinical features that would lead to a biopsy versus an alternative treatment.

Reading:

- *Andrews' Diseases of the Skin, Clinical Dermatology*— Epidermal Nevi, Neoplasms, and Cysts.
- *Dermatology*—Sections: Neoplasms of the Skin: Principles of Tumor Biology and Pathogenesis of BCCs and SCCs. Actinic Keratosis, Basal Cell Carcinoma, and Squamous Cell Carcinoma.

Week 12: Seborrheic Keratosis, Epidermal Tumors, and Cysts—Understanding the differential diagnosis for the common seborrheic keratosis, melanoma, and non-melanoma skin cancer is integral in the day-to-day practice of dermatology. At the same time, understanding the common benign growths of the skin, such as epidermal cysts, as well as the unusual dermal tumors, such as Merkel cell carcinoma, can be daunting. The important requisite is to teach the findings and clues that should lead a provider to know when further testing is necessary, such as a biopsy or excision.

Reading:

- *Andrews' Diseases of the Skin, Clinical Dermatology*— Epidermal Nevi, Neoplasms, and Cysts.
- *Dermatology*—Sections: Neoplasms of the Skin. Cysts. Adnexal Neoplasms. Benign Adnexal Neoplasms.

Chapter 35
Kodachrome DDx Sessions

One of the techniques that helps garner a mentality of formulating differential diagnosis is similar to what our Dermatology chairman termed "Kodachrome sessions." They are sessions where images of conditions serve as a source of discussion. These are excellent modalities for teaching the terminology of dermatology through descriptive practice. In addition, this facilitates a mental approach for formulating a differential diagnosis.

When done properly, the session can be as quick as fifteen to twenty minutes.

In today's technologically advanced world, it is relatively easy to search the Internet for several photographic images that correspond to the topic of study for the week. The physician should place on his or her monitor screen a few images of the conditions being studied, and also several items in the differential diagnosis. Then, have your NP or PA describe the primary and secondary lesions they see.

It is essential to let them use their words—not yours. When we see small children learning to speak, sometimes a parent will say, "Use your words." And then the child must think about what he wants, speak what his is to say, and then he receives what he has requested.

This is the premise of the DDx sessions. Make the NP or PA speak what they see, so they learn to place proper descriptive terms in the medical encounter note. Do not let them off the hook by you being the one to describe all the lesions. Make them think about it.

As they become more proficient and understand the lesions/diagnostic entities, they will better be able to comprehend the educational material they are working on each week. Building the vocabulary allows for more rapid assimilation of diagnostic skills.

In summary, providers who improve their performance in these sessions:

- ✓ be able to communicate more accurately to you
- ✓ create clearer and more concise encounter notes (important since the encounter note is the practice's legal documentation)
- ✓ learn to think in a way that they formulate a differential rather than simply throw out a diagnosis

The last sentence bears repeating: Teach them to start thinking in a way they formulate a differential rather than simply throw out a diagnosis.

Make sure they have lists of differentials and can recite the common ones in the list. As their knowledge grows, they can add the list.

Remember that dermatology is like a new language, and this process is often slow and requires patience from the provider.

The DDx sessions can be even more powerful when you have more than one provider participating. If you have two NPs or PAs, the group dynamic can help gather more thoughts and points of view on specific lesions. Including more people often adds more entities to the differential diagnosis.

Overall, this exercise builds a stronger framework of dermatology knowledge and can be enhanced with greater participation.

Chapter 36
Basic List for Differential Diagnosis Sessions

The power to formulate a differential diagnosis creates a much more solid provider. This is why our Dermwise training system terms the differential diagnostic groupings "Power Categories."

These categories are a valuable method of evaluating patients. Providers are encouraged to memorize the list of common entities in each category. As their knowledge grows, they should add to the list in each category.

A brief overview of the Power Categories appears to the right.

An NP or a PA who memorizes this card—at a minimum, the

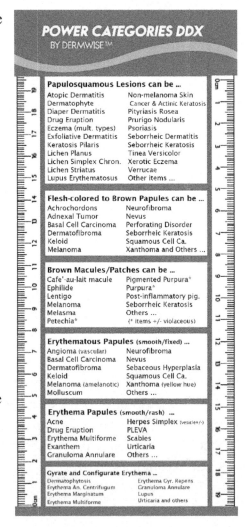

POWER CATEGORIES DDX
BY DERMWISE™

Papulosquamous Lesions can be ...

Atopic Dermatitis	Non-melanoma Skin
Dermatophyte	Cancer & Actinic Keratosis
Diaper Dermatitis	Pityriasis Rosea
Drug Eruption	Prurigo Nodularis
Eczema (mult. types)	Psoriasis
Exfoliative Dermatitis	Seborrheic Dermatitis
Keratosis Pilaris	Seborrheic Keratosis
Lichen Planus	Tinea Versicolor
Lichen Simplex Chron.	Xerotic Eczema
Lichen Striatus	Verrucae
Lupus Erythematosus	Other items ...

Flesh-colored to Brown Papules can be ...

Achrochordons	Neurofibroma
Adnexal Tumor	Nevus
Basal Cell Carcinoma	Perforating Disorder
Dermatofibroma	Seborrheic Keratosis
Keloid	Squamous Cell Ca.
Melanoma	Xanthoma and Others ...

Brown Macules/Patches can be ...

Cafe'-au-lait macule	Pigmented Purpura⁺
Ephilide	Purpura⁺
Lentigo	Post-inflammatory pig.
Melanoma	Seborrheic Keratosis
Melasma	Others ...
Petechia*	(* items +/- violaceous)

Erythematous Papules (smooth/fixed) ...

Angioma (vascular)	Neurofibroma
Basal Cell Carcinoma	Nevus
Dermatofibroma	Sebaceous Hyperplasia
Keloid	Squamous Cell Ca.
Melanoma (amelanotic)	Xanthoma (yellow hue)
Molluscum	Others ...

Erythema Papules (smooth/rash) ...

Acne	Herpes Simplex (vesicle+/-)
Drug Eruption	PLEVA
Erythema Multiforme	Scabies
Exanthem	Urticaria
Granuloma Annulare	Others ...

Gyrate and Configurate Erythema ...

Dermatophytosis	Erythema Gyr. Repens
Erythema An. Centrifugum	Granuloma Annulare
Erythema Marginatum	Lupus
Erythema Multiforme	Urticaria and others

papulosquamous category—early in the training often has a stronger path to success.

Chapter 37
"Google It"

One of the candidates we talked with while interviewing to fill an NP/PA position in our office shared a frustration. Even though he had been a PA for eleven years, he wanted to be in a location where the supervising physician was engaged.

I questioned him further. He said that at his previous job he had worked fairly autonomously, and once every few weeks (he perceived this was the minimum legal amount of time required), the supervising physician flew in his private plane to visit his remote clinic. He would spend part of a day (mostly reviewing pathology, which he read himself), and then leave. When the PA brought up medical questions, he told me, he was instructed to "Google it."

When I was a first-year dermatology resident, a senior resident, Dr. Dan Wall, told me in clinic that he and a volunteer faculty member, Dr. James Ertle, had just seen a patient who "had classic distribution and symptoms of dermatitis herpetiformis." I can remember like it was yesterday just how overwhelming dermatology felt at the time. It was hard the first few months to get a handle on atopic dermatitis, psoriasis, and the common conditions. This new diagnosis of dermatitis herpetiformis was not something I was familiar with.

Not to let a learning opportunity go by, I asked Dr. Ertle what the locations were that Dan was talking about. A man of few words, he merely stated it was the typical distribution.

As I learned later, he was so good-natured that I could have exposed my ignorance further and he would have gladly explained the distribution. But at the time, yikes, I felt like a fool for asking. I took off like a dog with my tail between my legs, went home that night, and read about dermatitis herpetiformis.

Now, I gradually got to know Dr. Ertle better. I have to say that he never had a negative interaction with a single person, and he volunteered every Tuesday of his life for the residents' education. All unpaid, I might add. He won faculty member of the year, and has been honored in many venues. There is no finer person that I know of.

That being said, I found my initial, brief interaction with him intimidating. However, it taught me to learn what I could learn, and then ask questions.

In other words, don't ask the question you should have looked up. Ask the questions you have after you looked up the topic.

This is a point that can help your NP or PA. The supervising physician role is to facilitate, help, and guide them. At the same time, they have a responsibility and an obligation to be students of the specialty. If all they learn is what we see and talk about in the clinic, they might look good and smooth at first, but they will have no depth to their dermatology skill set.

The depth and fund of knowledge is what helps keep them and their patients out of trouble. So, NP and PA providers should be taught that they must read and learn to research the conditions they see.

It is best to encourage them to get their bearings about the diagnosis and literature—if possible, before asking questions. Obviously, this is for instances when there is time to do so.

NP and PAs need to be trained to think, not just pull on the clinic experiences they have "seen" in clinic. It is the same responsibility physicians have, and it must be encouraged, nurtured, and grown in the NP or PA.

An effective teaching strategy I have found is this: If the question about a patient is not one that requires an immediate response, I ask them to write up the question and send it to me (we have an electronic record with a messaging system). For any question they send, they are encouraged to research the condition. Then, after they have looked up the topic, we meet to go over the possible solutions and determine the best one.

In this regard, they are growing with each question. At times, we both learn something.

Also, when I am asked a question about an abnormal lab or unusual finding, my reply might be, "What does Wolverton's *Comprehensive Dermatologic Drug Therapy* say?" Rather than give the answer, ask them to research for more information. Then together a decision can be made.

There are other modalities to teach, and this pattern is one that I personally have found helps myself and our providers to grow together in knowledge. In the long run, a supervising physician and their NP or PA are collaborating in the care of patients. Arming the NP or PA with the skill set to answer some of their own questions helps them become a more complete provider.

Self-education is critical in today's ever-expanding world of knowledge. Teaching a provider *how* to learn is, at times, more important than teaching them what is seen in the clinic. Find a way to get your provider to become engaged, hone their critical-thinking skills, and you will improve the quality of care in your practice.

Chapter 38
How Do Humans Remember Best?

As we train new hires, it might be helpful for us to understand what scientists label as "keys to learning." At times, it is presumed that a new topic should just be assimilated rapidly and mastered. Unfortunately, learning does not work this way for most people.

As touched on previously, supervising physicians sometimes forget it took a formal residency, grand round sessions, research projects, preparing lectures, attending lectures, seeing many, many patients, and much more over years (after four years of medical school, no less) to attain proficiency in their field. Sometimes it even took a few years after completion of residency to feel like they had a grasp on their specialty.

At the same time, while all of the knowledge was pushed on resident physicians, they were under the threat of having to pass a board specialty exam.

Success is necessary for a physician to be able to practice and pay back loans.

The pressure is not quite the same for an NP or a PA to find success in specialty practice. And in many cases, supervising physicians try to train their new hire by clinical osmosis. By this I mean they tote them around clinic and tell them a few pearls over the course of the day. No examinations, lectures, research projects, presentations, or any of the other items that were critical in the physician's training and subsequent specialization are utilized.

Most people grasp new material best when their instructor or mentor employ as many techniques to maximize learning as possible.

As I touched on previously, in the book *Accelerated Learning* by Colin Rose, the scientific basis for learning is reviewed. Studies are used to back the claims for the most efficient manner in learning. Being aware of some of these techniques is helpful.

The way time is spent and the distribution of information can have an enormous impact on learning.

- Rose indicated psychologists have found if someone takes 30 minutes of learning material and breaks it up into two days, the material can be learned in only 22 minutes, which is a 30 percent savings.
- Plus, if material is presented two times with a short time between the reviews, it can be retained more readily.
- Also, active involvement is more helpful than passive learning. In fact, the more involved a person is in learning (i.e., organizing topics themselves, looking up factors in journals and books to corroborate, etc.) the deeper the learning.
- When people learn a mental map, and can add to it in a manner in which they understand connections or principles involved, the subject is given meaning and personal relevance. This can then tie together items of significance by allowing the mind to see them as emotionally relevant.
- In addition to these findings, it has been shown the first items of a lesson (the primacy effect) and the last items of it (the recency effect) are most easily recalled.

In our training, we regularly incorporate each of the above items into the learning program. It is how humans remember best.

When we understand how the mind performs optimally, methods can be utilized to build a training system that fosters rapid learning and retention. The goal of training is competency as fast as possible. Employing some of these advanced learning and memory techniques help expedite proficiency.

The following combination for our new NP or PA hires has proven extremely efficient and successful.

1) Weekly Dermwise Quick Start Online Dermatology Training system—video modules and required reading.
2) Weekly meetings with a supervising physician to review content and important points.
3) Weekly differential diagnostic (DDx) sessions.
4) Weekly examinations through the Dermwise Training system.

All of the above can be combined with your NP or PA's involvement in the care of as many patients as possible, in order to maximize their exposure and clinical experience.

Dermwise Training utilizes and incorporates many of the advanced learning techniques. When you combine this with a weekly schedule as described, you are utilizing and integrating one of the most efficient training processes available. At the same time, the dermatologist is being exceptionally efficient with his or her time.

Part Four

Integration of an NP or a PA

Chapter 39
Why the Integration of Your
NP or PA Is So Important

If a business loses a customer, it is said to cost five times as much to replace them with a new customer than to keep the original customer happy.

As noted earlier in the book, at Disney World and Disneyland, each visitor/tourist is treated as a guest, and in turn, people willingly pay for what they deem is a wonderful experience. Many visitors save for an entire year or more to partake in this endeavor. The environment, service, and quality are so distinctive that people feel the experience outweighs the cost.

Why is this important? Because it demonstrates the psyche of the human mind. If the environment, service, and overall experience are spectacular, then price is less of an issue.

The Disney experience reminds me of an example in our field, presented at the American Academy of Dermatology meetings, where a practice treated cosmetic patients like they were in a five-star resort. One of the services they provided was to have a member of the medical team bring in a warm towel on a silver platter for each cosmetic patient before they received their injection.

I can only imagine the first time someone experiences this treatment, especially after being herded through like cattle at the office down the street. The likelihood of this practice's patient sharing their experience with others is almost certainly much higher than the provider who simply does a great job injecting the filler or botulinum toxin.

Retention of customers or clients by offering quality service—or even stellar service—is paramount to the viability of any business, or in our case, the practice.

How do we retain clients? It begins (and ends) with providing trustworthy, quality service, and it has everything to do with relationships.

Thus, a patient is really a client, someone who has the choice to go elsewhere.

Each happy client brings lifetime value to a practice. This means that over the course of the relationship, the patient (if kept happy) will return multiple times, creating a profit that is equal to the total profit of all the visits, not simply one visit.

In many businesses, the lifetime value of clients is estimated to be as great or greater than seven times the original amount of profit earned on one visit. For a patient who comes in for repeated cosmetic procedures, has actinic keratosis required to be treated repeatedly, or ends up with multiple skin cancers, the value over years can be dramatically higher.

Lifetime value also expands as clients refer friends and family to the business or practice. Then each of those friends and family members have lifetime value as well.

Understanding retention of patients and the value of each patient encounter is all-important when integrating and transitioning care for your established patients to your NP or PA. The patient must deem his or her experience with the NP or PA as worthy of returning for future visits, or else the practice risks losing the lifetime value of the patient, as well as the value of the friends and family members the patient would otherwise refer.

We must make every effort to have a highly trained NP or PA who is competent in knowledge and in effective communication. For this to occur, the providers of a practice must be educated, trained, and integrated exceptionally well.

Chapter 40
Tips for Integration of Your Provider with Staff and Patients

The NP or PA integration must fit the culture of yourself, your staff, and the new provider. This means, at the onset of hiring, it is best to explain what is expected and set reasonable goals.

Your provider integration must also fit the expectations of your patients. Once your administrative staff and medical support staff understand the role of your NP or PA, the next strategy to consider is how to gain patient acceptance.

Patient acceptance of non-physician providers is steadily on the rise. It is important to educate patients on your NP or PA, including what an NP or a PA is, the training they have done before joining your practice, the training they have undergone after joining your practice, and/or the duration of employment or experience in dermatology.

At our office, the Dermwise training system is a staple of new hires. Highlighting this can provide reassurance to our patients that there is a high standard which our NPs and PAs uphold. Sharing this information with the patients sets up the expectations of quality care and reassures them. (In addition, assessing the knowledge of the provider with examinations (written or verbal) to evaluate competency can help you to understand if the NP or PA is ready for the responsibility given.)

There are many ways to educate your patients about what an NP or a PA has to offer. A choreographed effort to build trust and highlight the time and effort you have invested in this person should be in place. This includes website information, phone scripts, offering appointments by medical staff, pre-appointment letters or e-mails, placement of signage and other informational materials (such as brochures or biography sheets—see next chapter) in the office and exam rooms, signage on paperwork, discussion by medical staff, and much more.

Some of the techniques used to educate patients about an NP or a PA can effectively be used as an opportunity to market the exceptional quality of care your team provides. The informational materials you furnish are a vote of confidence for the NP or PA.

Having patients see the NP or PA one time and then the dermatologists the next time, or some other rotating schedule, can ensure that the high level of care you expect for your patients is being carried out. A rotating pattern is common for many dermatologists, who indicate that they like to see their patients themselves no less than once a year.

Employing some form of a team approach can also ensure your patients are getting the best care possible. The more qualified eyes, hands, and brains handling treatment and patient care, the better.

If you employ a rotation of appointments, it is best to tell your patients so they know what to expect. Also let them know you are available for questions if your NP or PA has questions or concerns about their care. In busy practices, like most of us have, you may be able to delegate to your medical assistants or nursing staff the explanation of how the scheduling with the NP or PA integrates with their care. If you are delegating any discussion of this nature, it would be advisable to write down what you expect each patient to be told in order to formulate a script that can be repeated the way you want it.

Take the time to share with your patients who your NP or PA is, the benefits of their involvement in their care, and provide education regarding their competency. These steps are essential to continuing the strong bond you have established with your patients. Successful integration can have a resounding effect on your practice growth.

Chapter 41
Biography Sheets

A simple method to introduce and market your NP or PA is to create a laminated biography sheet to be placed in all exam rooms used by the provider.

In our office, on the back side of this sheet, we place a description of what a nurse practitioner or physician assistant is, how they work with physicians, and that they can write prescriptions and perform procedures, much like the dermatologist.

On the front side, a professional biography is written for the NP or PA. Information detailing education, prior experience, and location are customary. As stated in the previous chapter, this is an opportunity to feature the dermatology training the provider has had before joining your practice, or the education you have provided them since they were brought on board.

The ideal scenario is for the information to reassure patients they have made a wise decision with your practice and are secure in the capable hands of your NP or PA.

From a human relations standpoint (remember, relationships are all-important), patients also like to feel they have familiarity and can identify with their provider. Adding a photo can reassure them before they meet the provider in person. Also adding information about other qualifications/education, family, and hobbies can help form a bond with patients.

As noted in the previous chapter, biography sheets can be placed in the waiting room, in the exam rooms the NP or PA are working out of, and in procedure rooms so that patients may read it when waiting to be seen. Invariably, the patients have to wait a few minutes in the exam room, and this is a great time for them to read about their provider.

You can also have your medical assistants hand the biography sheet to the patient and ask that they read it while they wait.

It is surprising how many patients will state they appreciate learning about the education or capability of the provider they are seeing. This component can be highly helpful in gaining acceptance for the seeing and NP or PA rather than the dermatologist.

It is best if the biography sheets look to be of superior professional quality. A high-quality local print shop can do this if you or your staff do not have the capability. They are well worth the investment.

If laminated, the form can last quite some time and stand up to frequent handling.

It is thus advised that you make a laminated biography sheet for your NP or PA, which educates patients and shares the human qualities of the provider. Professional appearing and laminated, this tool can stand the test of time and be a quiet workhorse in gaining patient acceptance. You will be amazed at how many patients appreciate the biography sheet.

Biography Sample

Meet our Physician Assistant:
 John Doe, PA-C

John has been a part of the ABC Dermatology Practice since 20XX. He grew up in (town, state), where he graduated valedictorian of his high school class. After high school, John earned a bachelor's degree in biology from (name) University. He had always dreamed of working with patients in a medical setting, so he went on to earn his master's degree at (name of) University in Physician Assistant Studies.

John brings with him a vast level of education and experience. In addition, he has trained under the guidance of highly trained and experienced dermatologist Dr. Supervisor of ABC Dermatology for/since (time/date) to ensure he will provide the best possible care for his patients.

He is a member of the American Academy of Physician Assistants (AAPA), the State Academy of Physician Assistants (SAPA), and the Society of Dermatology Physician Assistants (SDPA).

When John is not in the office, he enjoys spending time with his wife and two sons, and their friends, and taking long walks in the park with Max, his Labrador Retriever. He also enjoys gardening, fishing, running, and golf.

Review of the Biography Sample

You will notice the first two paragraphs give a brief synopsis of the PA. It is important to have a concise, clear image a patient can take from this information. This means the biography should provide answers to questions a patient may have in mind about their provider. Any research, special interests, or advanced training should be mentioned.

The third paragraph identifies what societies, and activities related to the practice of his specialty, are involved. Not sharing enough about the accomplishments of the provider is a mistake many medical practices make. Do not assume the patients know or have researched online before the appointment. Featuring attributes in this section assists credibility and is valued by the average patient.

The final paragraph highlights some personal details, including family, pets, and social activities. Particulars about any awards, notable positions held, or non-medical involvement can be placed here also. It is common for these items to allow for a social connection.

The ability to see a provider as a human who has similar interests or life experiences can facilitate a relationship bond. We had one provider who became an Eagle Scout and another who was a former Marine. Patients expressed a strong affinity for providers who connected with them because of these factors.

Personal Connections Matter

If you are not sharing something personal about yourself or your NP/PA on your marketing material, you would be amazed at how a little information of this type can resonate and captivate your patient base. It does not have to be your most intimate activities, but maybe that you like to exercise at the gym, grew up on a farm, took a gardening class, worked at a drug store in high school, or some other point of potential mutual interest.

That connection allows patients to feel like they have a commonality. Interestingly, it can enable them to overcome barriers that might cause anxiety or fear of their appointments. We often see people who have not been to a doctor in years, and at times the human relationship connection can help facilitate a willingness to treat a medical condition in need of care.

Patients often look at providers as authorities, even as celebrities, of sorts. If they run into you at the store, they may very well tell their spouse or friends they saw you in the store and that you said hello. A willingness for a provider to share something personal about themselves can help create an opening for a connection beyond what can be felt as the cold, sterile medical environment. The human connection is important for building trust and an ongoing relationship.

Understanding the psychology of yourself, what you are willing to share, and what boundaries you and your NP or PA would like upheld, is key. At the same time, allowing patients to see their providers as human can be bountifully rewarding to both the patients and the providers.

Physician Assistant Description Sample

The back of the biography sheet can have what you would like on it, keeping in mind it is an opportunity to educate and reassure patients about the provider they are seeing. It can be tailored to fit what you would like to highlight about your NP or PA.

An example of the back side of a biography sheet is as follows.

What is a Physician Assistant?

PAs work in concert with physicians, complementing the physician's ability to deliver a comprehensive range of medical services. PAs' rigorous education, versatility, and commitment to individualized treatment help physicians function more efficiently and enhance continuity of health care.

—American Academy of Physician Assistants

The following might be an alternative.

What is a Dermatology Physician Assistant?

Physician assistants (PAs) in dermatology evaluate, diagnose, and treat a broad variety of conditions that are treated both medically and surgically.

They also perform screening exams, preventive care, and education for dermatologic patients and families.

Building on their primary-care training and experience, PAs are trained in dermatology in a variety of ways. Most dermatology PAs are trained in the clinic by the collaborating dermatologist, and together the physician-PA team will decide the practice style, collaboration agreement, and delegation of services that they find appropriate for their practice.

Most PAs work autonomously within a dermatology office, much like a staff dermatologist seeing a wide range of medical, surgical, and cosmetic patients, but always with the support of a board-certified or board-eligible dermatologist.

PAs get additional education through their required CME (continuing medical education) hours, attendance at AAD (American Academy of Dermatology), SDPA (Society of Dermatology Physician Assistants), and other dermatology-based conferences, tumor boards, dermatology grand rounds, and self-study courses. Some PAs hold master's degrees in PA studies, with a concentration in dermatology.

—Society of Dermatology Physician Assistants
(www.dermpa.org, 2017)

Nurse Practitioner Description Sample

The back of the biography sheet can read something like the following for your nurse practitioner.

What is a Nurse Practitioner?

Nurse practitioners (NPs) are medical clinicians that hold master's degrees or doctoral degrees, and have advanced clinical training beyond their initial professional nurse preparation.

Didactic and clinical courses prepare these professionals with specialized knowledge and clinical competency to practice in primary care, acute care, long-term health care settings, and with advanced training in specialty clinics such as our dermatology office.

NPs are quickly becoming the health partner of choice for millions of Americans. As clinicians that blend clinical expertise in diagnosing and treating health conditions with an added emphasis on disease prevention and health management, NPs bring a comprehensive perspective to health care.

Americans make over 916 million visits to NPs every year.

—American Association of Nurse Practitioners

The back of the biography sheet is an excellent place to share how your NP or PA works with you in your clinic or has been educated. This is an opportunity to educate those who have a limited knowledge of NP and PAs regarding their capabilities, education, and role. At the same time, it is an excellent occasion to share what sets your NP or PA apart from the competition.

For our practice, we utilize the Dermwise Quick Start Online Training System as a distinguishing factor. The biography sheet is an excellent place to share about this training, the rigors of the educational process, and how our NP or PA works with me in the clinic.

An example of the back side of a biography sheet is as follows.

What is a Dermatology Physician Assistant?

Physician assistants (PAs) in dermatology evaluate, diagnose, and treat a broad variety of conditions, both medically and surgically. PAs can perform skin cancer screening exams, prescribe medications, perform biopsies, and administer cryosurgery (freezing or liquid nitrogen).

Most dermatology PAs are extensively trained in the clinic by the collaborating dermatologist, and together the physician-PA team decide the practice style, collaboration agreement, and delegation of services appropriate for their practice.

Most PAs work autonomously within a dermatology office, seeing a wide range of medical, surgical, and cosmetic patients, but always with the support of a board-certified or board-eligible dermatologist.

Each PA has graduated with a master's degree and holds a license to practice medicine. They get additional education through CME (continuing medical education) hours, attendance at AAD (American

---

Academy of Dermatology), and other dermatology-based conferences.

At our practice (or insert practice name), our PAs are put through the rigorous Dermwise Online Training System. This involves advanced training in dermatology and requires examinations to verify mastery of content. In addition to the intense didactic education with Dermwise, our PA sees every new patient and new diagnosis with our dermatologist until competency is verified.

At (insert practice name), patient care is our highest priority, and our PAs are trained at the highest level possible.

A customized biography sheet is thus a strong educational tool that can not only reassure and educate patients, but also distinguish your NP or PA (as well as your practice) from your competition. Take the time to build this tool, and you will reap the benefits for years to come.

Chapter 42
Promotion by Website

In today's world, a great number of patients utilize the Internet for finding a provider, learning about their provider, and locating the clinic. An up-to-date website is a sign of a modern and progressive practice, and it draws many new patients to the office.

Adding the biography sheet's information about the NP or PA to the website is a must. This can be a powerful opportunity to create a bond before the patient arrives. The information can easily be updated if the NP or PA gains certifications, education, or lectures the community.

The website is also a great place to utilize links to national organizations that add credibility and serve as a third-party endorsement and validation, such as listing membership to Society of Dermatology Physician Assistants.

If your state or city has a dermatology society, this is another place to have the NP or PA join. From a prospective patient's viewpoint, it is nice to find your provider in a list of dermatology specialists in the area. The value in letting the world know your provider is a member cannot be underscored enough.

In addition, testimonials contributed by colleagues and/or happy patients of the NP or PA can be placed on the website. These third-party endorsements are typically seen as independent sources reassuring prospective patients of the quality of experience and care the NP or PA provides. What someone says about the provider can be much more trusted and valuable than what the practice can state.

All of these points are reminders that practices in today's modern world must consider utilizing the power of the Web to the practice's advantage. Address concerns patients might have about abilities of their provider, training they have, and quality of care. In this manner, the website can and should be a strong ally to the practice.

Chapter 43
Personal Introduction by the Supervising Physician

Another method (which may actually be one of the best) to aid in patient acceptance of your NP or PA is a personal introduction from the supervising physician. One way in which this can occur is when the supervising physician is transferring care to the NP or PA.

For example, a patient on the dermatologist's schedule has a verrucae, which requires a series treatment plan (specifically, ongoing treatments for three to four months), so the patient will return in a few weeks. If the supervising physician does not have an opening, he or she may explain to the patient that their next follow-up appointment is being transitioned to the NP or PA, and what the patient should expect.

Then the physician can bring the NP or PA into the exam room and provide a personal introduction, so the patient meets the provider they will see at the next visit.

For the sake of time, the physician may mention the introduction during the visit, the medical assistant can take the cue, go get the NP or PA, and have them ready to introduce as the visit winds down.

The introduction can also be accomplished when the NP or PA is in the early training phase (shadowing), whereby they may already be in the room with the physician at the appointment.

Here is an example of what the supervising physician might say. "Ms. Jones, I believe you have a severe case of seborrheic dermatitis. My next follow-up appointment is not available for a couple of months. I would like for John, my physician assistant, to see you in the next two weeks, to make sure you have responded to the treatment as expected. This is John, and he will take excellent care of you."

In addition to the personal introduction, you can explain to John in front of the patient what course of treatment you have decided on for Ms. Jones, what the next step would be if she responds well, and what the next step would be if she does not respond well. This information should also be documented in the patient's chart.

The patient then sees the supervising physician involvement in the problem and understands the dermatologist is the leader and chief strategist in their care.

The synergy created by this interaction can help facilitate a strong bond with the patient and both the supervising physician and the NP or PA.

A human-relations tactic worth mentioning in this scenario is to consider letting the patient know that if they prefer to follow up with the physician, this is fine, though the next appointment may be booked out a bit farther. The opportunity to choose allows the patient to be given the respect they often appreciate in this situation. The choice proposition can yield a higher buy-in for the situation as well.

Chapter 44
Letter to Patients Introducing the NP or PA

Another wonderful way to facilitate integration and acceptance of the NP or PA is to provide the patients who will see them with a letter of introduction. This method can create awareness of the capabilities of the provider they will see, reiterate competency, and provide reassurances that the patient is in capable hands.

In an ideal scenario, this would be done for every patient who will see the NP or PA—both new and existing patients. In the real world, the occurrence of this, if it happens at all, is often tied solely to new patients of the practice. It is not uncommon for progressive practices to send patients information about their first-time visit to the practice, though you may also want to consider sending the letter to all patients the provider will care for.

The first-time introduction letter is an outstanding way to market the practice, detail the services offered, and establish the reputation (and value) of the NP or PA.

The primary concept is to provide reassurances the patient has made the right choice in selecting your practice. The second important point is to start a foundation of trust in the relationship with the NP or PA, in addition to building trust in the practice.

The introduction letter would ideally be written by the supervising physician. In larger practices, alternatives can include the founding partner, marketing director, or office manager. Whomever you select to write the letter, make sure they meet the goals of reassuring correct choice and establishing, or deepening, rapport with the patient.

An example of a letter of this type follows.

Dear Ms. New Patient,

Thank you for scheduling an appointment at ABC Dermatology. Our number one priority is to provide you with the best possible care for you and your skin.

We see that you have scheduled to see our dermatology physician assistant, John Doe, PA-C. We would like to thank you and provide you with some brief information regarding what a physician assistant is, as well as the benefits of seeing John in the near future.

What is a physician assistant?

A dermatology physician assistant (PA) is a highly trained medical provider who holds a master's degree in physician assistant studies. PAs see a wide range of patients and are able to diagnose and treat common dermatologic conditions, order and interpret diagnostic tests, perform procedures, and prescribe medications.

Dr. Supervisor requires each of his PAs to complete rigorous online dermatology educational courses, including examinations. Dr. Supervisor is confident in the ability of his PA and can ensure that you are in good hands.

Why am I seeing a PA instead of Dr. Supervisor?

You always have the choice to see Dr. Supervisor, if you would prefer. However, Dr. Supervisor's schedule is often booked out several months, and it can take longer for you to get in to see him/her. Seeing our dermatology-trained PA allows you to have easier access to high-quality dermatology care and rapid follow-up.

If you prefer to reschedule your appointment to see Dr. Supervisor, please contact our office. You always have this choice.

For more detailed information about the PA you are scheduled with, please see below *(or you could direct them to your website)*.

John Doe, PA-C
(Insert John Doe's biography here.)

If you have any questions regarding your appointment, please do not hesitate to give us a call at XXX-XXX-XXXX. Our goal is to help you maintain healthy, beautiful skin.

For more information about our practice, please visit our website at www.examplewebsite.com.

Sincerely,
Practice Administrator

Note that the example above is designed to educate about what a physician assistant is and can do. This is helpful if the physician assistant is a new concept for your practice, and your patients might benefit from learning what a PA is and what to expect.

However, if your practice has an NP or a PA already and/or the patients in your region are familiar with the NP and/or PA model of practice, you can tailor this letter to educate more specifically about the provider. The key in this scenario is to provide a synopsis and an endorsement that help build the relationship between the provider and your patients.

If you elect to send a welcome packet with a letter, it is ideal to send these letters to patients at least one week before the patient is scheduled, in case a change in appointment type is necessary.

A personal letter that appears to be written by the supervising physician introducing the NP or PA can also help enhance patient confidence in their ability. In addition, this reminds patients that they can always see the doctor if they wish, a powerful tool for gaining patient acceptance.

You can also speak to your web services or IT staff member to determine if this type of information can be sent out in an e-mail maintaining HIPAA compliance. The patient portal can also provide information to help navigate patients to the content you would like them to read.

See another example of an introduction letter from a supervising physician, below.

Hello, My Friend,

I want to personally thank you for choosing our practice at ABC Dermatology. We appreciate the opportunity to care for you. We have you scheduled for a visit soon with our physician assistant, John Doe, PA-C.

Before your visit, I would like to share a bit about what a physician assistant is and provide background

---

on John.

Physician assistants, commonly referred to as PAs, have training beyond a four-year degree, like nurse practitioners. A PA holds a master's degree. When certified and licensed like John, they can see patients, perform procedures, and write prescriptions. His care is administered under my supervision, and I review his charts and plans regularly.

I have chosen to have a physician assistant because this allows our patients to have access to a highly trained dermatology-trained provider quickly. Most of the time you will be able to get appointments without much wait time by utilizing our PA. This can make a big difference in how soon you feel better if you have a problem.

It is our priority that you have a positive experience seeing a provider you are comfortable with. John is an exceptional provider who has a high commitment to quality care. He has also been through my rigorous training program, including required dermatology reading, lectures, and examinations.

From early on in his training with me until now, he has been able to accurately diagnose and expertly develop treatment plans. I know he is quite capable, and you are in excellent hands. Should he have any questions at all about your care, he can easily contact me.

For your convenience, we have additional practice information available on our website at www.yourwebsitehere.com.

If, for any reason, you would rather see only myself as

the doctor, please call immediately and ask our scheduling staff to move your appointment back to a time when I am available. We look forward to seeing you, and thank you for being part of our dermatology family.   Sincerely,

Dr. Iam Supervisor

In our practice, we have a specific introduction letter tailored for an NP and a different letter for the PA. Adding to the letter that the provider has gone through the Dermwise Online Training Program provides credibility that a dermatology-specific educational system has been utilized. At the same time, some patients will look up the Dermwise website and find reassurance that their provider has this specific dermatology training. Regardless of how you educate your provider, share the education and qualifications as they aid credibility for your NP or PA.

An introduction letter to the practice for new patients, or a letter to those seeing only the NP or PA, can be a solid investment in establishing expectations and the patient-provider relationship. This letter is an investment in the success of your provider.

Chapter 45
Presentations in the Waiting Room

Today, there are so many technological avenues for getting information out to patients, that the only limit is our own time and creativity. Developing videos, social media posts, and similar marketing techniques are adjuvants to the progressive business model. The point of these strategies is to engage the patient and become one of the voices they respect and listen to.

With this in mind, another option for informing and educating your patients about a new NP or PA in your practice is through presentations that run periodically in your office.

When a patient is in the waiting room, they are a captive audience. Some practices take advantage of this by deploying marketing videos about their cosmetic services. This same premise can be utilized to educate patients about the field of nurse practitioners and physician assistants.

A simple presentation may contain information on what an NP or a PA is, the benefit of seeing one in your office, and may remind patients that they can always see the doctor if they choose.

A patient who has had to wait for months to see the dermatology physician might like the opportunity to choose a faster route. This is particularly the case if the patient feels that their issue could have been capably handled by an NP or a PA, who was handpicked and trained by the physician they trust. Marketing material educating them of the possible choice can be invaluable.

There are many different ways in which you can utilize this tool, and it can be crafted to fit your practice's needs and ability.

It does not take a rocket scientist to create a presentation that contains the pertinent information about your specific NP or PA, as this can be easily done in a PowerPoint format. This can then be exported as video file, which can be played in the waiting room or exam room. It can be intermixed with other information the practice would like to use as marketing.

These presentations can be designed to play on a TV in the waiting room or engineered to loop on computers in the waiting room or exam rooms. Such presentations, if done properly, can capture the patient's interest and thus reduce the frustration of a long wait time.

This idea has the potential to be molded to fit into your practice however you see fit. When this modality is deployed, it can perform an educational and marketing role every minute the practice doors are open. When it is designed well, patients leave the practice feeling more certain about their care and more positive about the provider.

Chapter 46
The Magic Waiting Room Book

In addition to watching your insightful PowerPoint presentations, the patients in the waiting room should always have material to read and occupy their time, so as to make their wait as pleasurable as possible. Up-to-date magazines or other items to read are a staple of most waiting rooms. This is important, yet it is not enough.

The typical practice has a steady flow of new patients every week. The patients are often brought to the office by referral from a friend, referral from a physician, an advertisement, or a personal search to solve their problems. The amount of information they know about you, your team, or your practice is often small compared to what most practices assume these new patients know.

A method to provide subtle marketing and significant education to patients is through building a waiting room educational binder. This can provide information about the practice, the staff, the cosmetic services, and contain other useful educational material.

Note the word *educational*. When done properly, this book should inform new patients about what the practice would like them to know. The patient must feel they know the practice and team better after reviewing this.

Be aware: You should steer clear of creating a purely sales/marketing-focused book, to avoid "turning off" the patient.

A simple method we have found useful includes basic office or school supplies. Use a three-ring binder that is high quality, looks professional, and will represent the practice well. Aesthetics is key. Choose a binder color that matches the practice logo or waiting room colors, with a clear window on the front.

Design an attractive front cover with easy-to-read lettering that invites patients to read about the practice or team.

Inside, place clear plastic three-ring binder sheets that can be filled with letter-sized (8.5" x 11") paper.

On the paper inserts, provide a short synopsis of the practice and its philosophy. Placement of information as noted earlier in the book about "What is a Physician Assistant?" or "What is a Nurse Practitioner?" are great here. Direct this education to the patient who has not heard of NPs or PAs in health care. Follow this content with a page on how the NP or PA is used in your practice, and then provide biographical information about your NP or PA provider.

Add mini articles about causes and events the practice, physicians, and/or NP or PA support—such as annual free skin cancer screenings, support of charities, and social activities related to the practice. Provide answers to common questions patients may have.

Keep each section of writing brief and therefore inviting to read. The best manner of writing is in a warm, conversational tone.

Use captivating images and a lot of relaxing white space. When done in an aesthetically pleasing manner, possibly with the assistance of a graphic designer, the book becomes well read.

Though it seems rather simple and will not be read by all patients, this book can be one of the small yet powerful tools that helps create bonds with patients.

Strong bonds with patients are a key to them becoming strong referral resources.

Chapter 47
Phone Scripts That Provide an Outstanding Patient Experience

What is a phone script? It is a method to ensure that the team of an organization shares a common voice when communicating with customers, clients, or patients. This modality is used by most successful businesses in the United States and in many other countries as well.

The technique can vary, from specific words being spoken, to simply ensuring the same level of care and compassion comes across from the business.

As much as you and I may not like it, there is a sales psychology to handling phone calls. Reading a few books on sales or marketing can be insightful. Companies like Zappos spend weeks training their customer service representatives on how to provide exceptional service.

Medical practices would do themselves a great service by hiring and training staff who are consistent and represent the product well (which, in this case, is you and your provider(s)).

Having phone scripts in a medical practice are a method of providing support to the reception/scheduling staff and enhancing phone etiquette for your practice. If you have never heard your front-office staff answer the phone on a busy day, give it a try, but be prepared for a case of indigestion (or your eyes opened).

If your office is anything like most, the front-office staff finds that patients arrive in bunches and work comes in droves.

It is not uncommon to have multiple patients walk up to check in at the same time. The front-office staff is then required to decide who it is, what paperwork needs to be completed, if a new insurance card is needed, what copay or balance is to be collected, and if a patient is new they must input the demographic and insurance information.

All this has to be done before the patient can be brought to the examination room by the medical assistant.

Now, try asking this office person to answer the phone that has been ringing while they feel overwhelmed and a line of patients is looking on. What do you think the tone will be? It may not be pleasant. And the service the person receives on the phone or in front of them might not be the best.

There are several ways to handle these issues, and you might already have a system in place. The topic worth mentioning for consideration is how to control the results of the phone calls into your office. This is because, in health care, these calls have never been more important than when you have an NP or a PA on your team. It is imperative that patient calls are answered properly. This is the focal point where your team can provide an opportunity to promote and fill the schedule of your NP or PA.

Get Your Phones Answered Properly!

We may have seen the images of the receptionist chewing gum and doing their nails. Today, this person may not be smacking gum, but rather has the browser open to Facebook or a phone hidden on the lap, texting while taking a paycheck. This person's verbal cues will not reflect well on the practice.

How these phone calls are handled can have a tremendous impact on the image and quality that patients experience. Though many physicians leave this to their managers or receptionists, they shouldn't. This is as an integral part of the functioning of your business and should be treated with the respect it deserves.

Developing scripts that fit the personality of you and your practice is critical.

You might begin by asking all of your front-office staff to write down what they say to potential patients who call in. Ask the receptionists, and not the manager. The receptionists will likely tell you what they are saying, not what the manager would like them to say.

After you have obtained a copy, ask them to write down exactly what they hear others say when they answer the phone. Do this on two different days so you can evaluate consistency.

You can also ask the manager how he or she thinks the phones are being answered.

With this, you should have a basic assessment of the phone interactions.

If you want to take this another step further, there are companies offering their services that can record or listen in to phone calls as well as review any legal matters pertaining to the act of recording phone conversations.

The patients should experience consistent conversations with the reception/scheduling department.

At one point, my dentist recommended an endodontist for my root canal. He explained that I would get the root canal at the other office and then return to him afterward to complete the process.

Well, after I made the endodontist appointment, I called back to my dentist's office, as he had instructed, and let his receptionist know the date of the endodontist root canal.

She said I would have to call them back after the root canal so they could schedule me at that time.

After hanging up the phone, it dawned on me how difficult it would be for me to adjust my schedule on short notice like she asked. An hour or so later, I called back to my dentist's office and received a different receptionist, luckily. I asked if I could schedule my post-root canal completion, anticipating that I would have to tell my rationale in a long story.

This receptionist immediately told me the number of days after the root canal that were typically needed to be safe, and scheduled the appointment right then. No long story or justification on my end required.

In his office, the inconsistency in reception responses could very well drive away patients.

We must make sure our reception team is on the same page and represents the practice at the highest level possible. Patients judge the practice every day, and judge the front-line team first.

To begin, write phone scripts that address situations commonly encountered by those who answer the phone. The wording can be changed to fit what you feel is appropriate for your style. Make sure the culture you want will be represented on the phone. Share these with a few friends and get feedback. Let the reception team practice them several times a day. Get their buy-in by asking them to contribute suggestions to improve the scripts, and then review those. Make final scripts that can be shared easily.

Tell the team that each member is responsible for ensuring the rest of the team is following the scripts and solidifying they are all on the same page. It might be worth a try to make a game of it at first, by rewarding the one who speaks the script best or most consistently.

In this way, all receptionists will learn to provide consistently helpful patient-centered assistance.

Remind your staff that patients are often in need when they call in. Your staff must have empathy for the patients' situation and avoid simply blurting out, "The next available appointment is X weeks from now." Make sure the reception/scheduling team is aware that every call is important and that schedules should be filled.

Teach them to shine a positive light on your practice. For this, you might write a few lines of script that let the patient know they made a wise choice choosing your practice. A simple example might be, "Mike, I am glad you called, as we have excellent providers in our office who are experts at treating acne. Dr. Derm is booking out six weeks, and his physician assistant, Paul, who was personally trained by Dr. Derm, has an opening this Thursday. Would you like to be seen at the earlier appointment time?"

The opportunity to shine a positive light on the practice and the NP or PA can be relatively simple and, if handled properly, can provide a wonderful introduction for patients. Well-thought-out phone scripting provides an additional layer of successful integration for the NP or PA.

Chapter 48
Avoid the Rock Star Trap

In the medical office and exam rooms, there are as many ways to deal with patients as there are people. Why? Because each person is different, and they respond and react to the person they are dealing with. For this reason, many physicians who practice a long time get a group of raving fans. The patients are attracted to how the provider interacts with them and provides their medical care.

This process can lead to the fallacy of the rock-star, or movie-star, mentality. This celebrity mentality occurs when a provider gets surrounded by staff who are taught to say yes, yes, yes, when the provider speaks. Then the patients are only those who fit the right mold to mesh with the provider.

Too many of the people involved who follow and agree can grow some bad habits, which are not the healthiest for a business, a medical practice, or the provider.

Why is this issue worth discussing? Well for one thing, most physicians who are hiring an NP or a PA have been in practice long enough to feel they need help caring for their patient population. At the same time, they can be set in their ways, which can lead to a potential showdown if a new provider does not act like the supervising physician expects.

Thus, it is worth taking a long, hard look at the style of practice you employ each day. A true critical look can unmask some bad habits you may have that need to be broken before they are carried forward into the people you train the office.

Here are some signs that the rock-star/movie-star ego has snuck into your practice.

- Do the staff and physician find it easy to blame the disgruntled or unhappy patient?
- Does the physician easily get offended when questioned about care/diagnosis/treatment?
- Does the provider refuse to speak to an unhappy/dissatisfied patient?

If you answer yes to one of these questions, it is best to objectively evaluate your methods and make sure this is the style you want someone else to carry forward in your name. It is far easier to set a positive example at the outset than to tell someone they should do what you say, and not what you do.

When a practice has been busy and booked out for months, the customer service habits that were initially used to grow the business might backslide. A careful analysis of the current attitudes and demeanor of the providers and staff must be done. This is vital, because when a new provider is introduced, the level of customer service must be exceptional in order to fill the schedule, keep existing patients, and attain new patients.

It is wise to make sure superior customer service is expected and emphasized. Treating patients with empathy and as though they are appreciated is all-important. The patients who are listened to and feel genuinely cared for and respected will return and are more likely to refer.

As physicians, it is important to remember that you set the tone of your practice, each and every day, for the entire staff. Leaders lead by example. The smile and hello you give, and the compliment for a hard day's work or a task well done, are the positive ripples that get passed along to the patients.

These simple but highly influential behaviors performed by the supervising physician are going to be traits expected and expressed by the NP or PA.

If you have found yourself falling away from the customer service mentality of your practice, make sure you put emphasis on yourself and the team for excellence in this realm. As mentioned earlier in the book, Gandhi was credited with the quote, "Be the change you want to see in the world." Make your example one you want emulated by the NP or PA.

Chapter 49
Dealing with Humans
and Their Warts

Knowing that people are all different and come from every walk of life is paramount to professional success. Understanding human relations is crucial for the provider and underscores the interaction of the exam room and its impact on trust, compliance, and return visits.

When a medical professional learns about human papilloma virus and the ugly warts caused by it, an uncanny realization unfolds with time. The rough-textured plaque is a medical challenge. This is because the painful treatment with cryosurgery often takes multiple sessions. The topical creams used for treatment have few studies to validate their usage and can become a treatment failure. The list of potential treatments and negative consequences goes on.

The point is not that people are warts. The point is that when a medical condition has a plethora of treatment options, the chances are there is no *one* definitive method of treatment.

This same premise holds true for human relations. There is no one secret that creates a successful interaction with every patient. However, there are some time-tested truths each provider should review and revisit occasionally in order to remain grounded in interpersonal fundamentals.

Right before my second year of medical school, I had the good fortune of being able to take the Dale Carnegie Course, which touched on human relations. It was given to me as a gift from the course instructor, who felt that my father's help in selling out two classes in our home town many years before had been a great benefit to him.

Had he not given me a scholarship to the program after my father died, I likely would have never taken the course. I am so humbled to have been through the training and would recommend it to anyone. The experience and content is worth every penny.

That being said, most people will not invest their time in the course. So, the very least you can do is spend a small amount on Dale Carnegie's book *How to Win Friends and Influence People*. The parables are a bit dated, but the principles and content are timeless.

Mr. Carnegie described tools and techniques that are helpful in dealing with others, including some strategies that make sense for health care providers. Just a few of his many principles include the following.

- Be a good listener; encourage others to talk about themselves.
- Talk in terms of the other person's interests.
- Remember that a person's name is, to that person, the sweetest and most important sound in any language.
- Smile.

These and Mr. Carnegie's other principles can seem basic to some people but are well worth mentioning and reviewing. All too often health care professionals become so ingrained in learning the facts of their specialty that they forget the human element as part of the "art of medicine." It is worth making sure this is rekindled or is going strong for you and your NP or PA.

There is never a more important time to think about this than when a new provider is intently focused on learning a new specialty. It is in these moments that the NP or PA may need a little nudge to remember they are not only in the medical-result business but also in the relationship-building business. The provider who develops a grand following from patients is the one who garners respect medically *and* from a human-relations dynamic.

Encourage your NP or PA to value human relations in their medical care. Some simple techniques for implementing the principles of human relations can pay large dividends.

Make the patient feel important. This can be as simple as a formal introduction and offering of pleasantries to help break down the rush a patient feels from the provider. A casual "how are you doing?" can be enough in some instances. Also, make eye contact while conversing with them. This demonstrates a level of respect and shows the other person they are valuable.

Ask if a patient has plans for the upcoming weekend or holiday. Inquire about work, hobbies, and other topics of conversation you might have shared in the past and noted.

Make the effort to place in the medical record something personal about them, which later can be recalled and mentioned. This can show an empathetic component to their provider.

Many patients know very well that a provider might have looked in their chart to get reminders of their hobbies, employment, or other items of importance, but many appreciate the effort.

While I wrote this book, one of my patients offered to bring in pictures of his red 1934 Ford Street Rod, which he had been working on for eighteen years. This was initiated by the recall, mention of the topic, and genuine interest I had shown at prior visits. The bond created by discovering what someone else enjoys can be quite strong.

A strong relationship can yield better medical care. Patients are more inclined to keep follow-up visits if they feel they are more than a number or a disease. The patients are also more likely to be compliant if they know their provider truly cares for them. Trust and relationships matter. Teaching or reminding your NP or PA of this can help grow your practice.

Chapter 50
Your NP or PA:
When Do You Turn Them Loose?

The point at which you schedule patients for your new provider can vary as much as you care to imagine. As clearly noted throughout this book, one of the primary reasons many practices hire the NP or PA is due to the fact that patients have a long wait time to be seen. The schedule of the NP or PA is often more accommodating, at least at first, so they can see patients in more timely manner. This creates an opportunity for the practice to serve patients and fill the provider's schedule.

Scheduling, in many practices I have had the privilege of engaging with, include an initial shadowing phase. During this time, the NP or PA is utilized to either follow or share patients with the supervising physician.

Shadowing often includes time for the new hire to learn the office dynamics, including software or paper chart, how to record biopsies, instructions on after-care for cryosurgery, and other tasks they will perform or be responsible for.

During the shadow phase, the NP or PA often functions the way many first-year dermatology residents would function. They see the patient, present verbally to the supervising physician, and then the supervising physician goes into the room and sees the patient, re-eliciting a history and completing the office visit. The NP or PA then writes in the chart and completes the note, which the physician then cosigns. Thus, patients are seen by two providers for the duration of shadowing.

Again, this method seems fairly consistent with practices I have spoken to. The variable components are 1) When does the NP or PA take on a more independent role? and 2) How is that determined? The latter aspect of independence can be challenging to determine.

Many practices use a time limit, such as three, six, or twelve months before an NP or a PA who is new to the field may see new problems or patients. The new provider is thus expected to take on and manage the patients who are assigned to them after a certain time period. The challenge with a time-based approach is that it does not always take into account the knowledge necessary to function at the level expected. A dilemma is self-evident in this scenario.

Other practices set a certain number of patients with each diagnosis, and only let the NP or PA see those types of patients. This can help provide at least a basis for knowing there is a level of practical experience. The challenge with this quota-based system is there is no verification of knowledge with exams/testing. In addition, a provider may only gain the knowledge of what was seen in clinic rather than the breadth of knowledge necessary.

Still other practices use educational parameters, such as lectures, text reading, or online article review, to determine capability to see patients independently. This provides a didactic approach to the training of a new NP or PA. It can follow the system most recent graduates have utilized to perform their school work. The problem is that without examinations and clinical competency evaluations, this method can lead to false assumptions of capabilities.

A select few practices set up a *full-spectrum* system to employ clinical time frames with goals expected, a system to verify that new hires have:

- seen certain diagnostic entities multiple times before being "signed off" on
- a schedule for reading
- a didactic series of education
- examinations

The main reason many practices do not do all of these items is the effort and time required by the supervising physician to invest in the process.

Most likely, the full-spectrum system is what most supervising physicians would indicate is the favored method of training. At the same time, each physician who has employed an NP or a PA would state the individual being trained is different, and thus variations of the items noted are often required.

At the very least, a physician who has a general guideline of diagnostic entities expected to be seen, reading to be accomplished, time spent in didactic sessions on these specific entities, and ideally examinations of some form, will have the best results.

A plan on how to manage the training can be invaluable, if it is decided at the outset.

In our practice, I am a bit overbearing compared to what I hear from other physicians, but I want our reputation to be extremely high, and I am a bit compulsive about my involvement in the patients of our practice. For our new NP or PA, I try diligently to see every new problem and every new patient with them for one year, if they are directly out of school. Many physicians stop seeing every new patient and/or problem much sooner. You can select the time you are most comfortable with, based on the progression of your NP or PA.

Every new problem and every new patient seems a lot. In fact, it is. But what I have found is that my time in the room tends to diminish not too long after a well-managed training period, in large part because the new provider is doing the charting and patient education/counseling. Some of the procedures can be delegated as well, once competence is demonstrated during the training period.

A way to justify the supervising physician's time in the rooms is that most insurance carriers, including Medicare, will pay an NP or a PA 85 percent of the physician's fees unless the visit is "incident-to." This means the office can collect 15 percent more for the visit when the physician performs the history, exam, and creates the assessment and plan. This can be done efficiently as the new hire gains knowledge. Of note is that when guidelines are followed to maintain "incident-to" billing, the follow-up visit is permitted to be billed under the physician's fee schedule rather than at 85 percent of the physician's fee. Thus, in some cases where the criteria are met, two visits can gain 15 percent with only the first requiring the physician involvement.

Ultimately, the decision on how rapidly your NP or PA will see new problems and new patients without you depends on the varied components discussed here. Demonstration of competence and quality decisions are provider-dependent. Set up a system to train and manage your NP or PA, and you the practice will find a wonderful addition to the team.

Chapter 51
When I Turn Them Loose

After hiring a new NP or PA, my approach is rather hands-on. At first, I see every new patient and every new problem with the new NP or PA. To get their knowledge up to par, this is continued for one year in my practice. After completion of the Dermwise training and satisfactory demonstration of their knowledge and clinical skills, including procedural capabilities and management of diagnostic entities, they are allowed to see follow-ups with established problems only.

I am going to share a bit about how I have chosen to educate and manage our NPs and PAs, with some of the reasons behind the process.

As a new hire joins our practice, I take their success very seriously. Their education is a primary fundamental core, and they are informed they must take the Dermwise online training program (www.dermwise.com) at a rate of one module per week. This gives them 12 modules in 12 weeks. The training has required reading, exams, and a pattern that follows the reputable textbooks *Andrews' Diseases of the Skin*: *Clinical Dermatology* and Dr. Jean Bolognia's *Dermatology*.

The premise is laid out that a solid foundation of dermatology knowledge is a must, and the knowledge must be attained quickly.

Part of the reason for being stern and giving the 12-week limit is that the person who develops good habits and learns of expectations early on should be someone who can be held to a high standard for a career.

In addition, the training is completed before the conclusion of their 90-day probationary period.

In some states, deciding whether to maintain or sever ties in an employment relationship before the 90 days is completed is important. It is best to look into your state laws or contact your lawyer. One fact to remind yourself, though, is if you have a reputation for your practice to uphold, you need a committed, hard-working provider who upholds the reputation of your practice alongside you. I recommend you encourage a strong education and hold people to it.

During the first three months of the training I provide, the NP or PA functions as a historian and a person who learns to present patients concisely. I see every patient with them, and they are scheduled for about one patient every thirty minutes. My philosophy, though, is not for them to find a wall to hold up in between the patients they present to me. They are expected to follow my every step when they are not with their own patient or working on charting. This means they may see four to six patients during each hour.

During this time, they are told to learn diagnosis, treatment plans, and watch how I interact with patients. It is amazing how many patients ask the same questions, provide similar histories, and bring in the same diagnostic entities. The NP or PA is to document a minimum number of acne, rosacea, verrucae, atopic dermatitis, psoriasis, and a few more entities they have seen.

The maintenance of me seeing every new problem and every new patient gives our care a team approach, yields physician-directed treatment plans, and provides patients a sense of physician involvement. In addition, visits of this type most often fall within the "incident-to" billing parameters, which maintains the physician fee schedule.

As the new skills develop, knowledge enhances, and confidence improves, I allow the new NP or PA to function a bit more independently.

The method and time dermatologists choose to invest in this process can vary dramatically. For some it is a matter of a few months, while others keep a tight control over the type of patients and situations they put their NP or PA into, for much longer. The pattern each dermatologist must choose is the one with which they feel most comfortable, and with which their patients receive outstanding care.

Chapter 52
The Difficult Patient

Recently, my nurse practitioner came to the administrator of our practice and told her that a patient he had seen became agitated and swore at him while stating he did not agree with the diagnosis he was given. The NP was not sure how he should have handled this and wanted the administrator's input.

Unfortunately, varied forms of "the challenging visit" happens frequently enough that the topic should be addressed. What is the issue? It can have multiple different forms, but the basic premise is that some unsatisfactory event occurs to cause a frustration in the quality of care, diagnosis rendered, treatment provided, fees required, or tardiness of appointment (running behind).

It can often be a sign of a lack of skills in handling the patient interaction and a lack of techniques or tools to facilitate a positive outcome.

One of our tasks as supervising physicians is to reduce complexities and simplify them, and these situations fall right within our wheelhouse.

Whether it is not agreeing with a diagnosis (lack of trust in care), running late in clinic, or simply handling a challenging situation with a patient, the NP or PA must be educated on the situation.

A challenge here is that most supervising physicians have less resistance, due to the fact that patients tend to hold "the doctor" in higher esteem. That component is one an NP or a PA must accept and work around. Also, many physicians have learned skills to cope with challenging patient interactions, which are second nature to them and often not viewed as a technique that can be taught.

Supplying our NP or PA with the tools to manage as many situations as possible helps them succeed.

Some of the common issues found in our practice will be reviewed below. Simply raising the level of awareness can help the practice run more smoothly, though others will arise in every practice.

Medical provider running late—I read once that a technique used in a chain restaurant was to acknowledge (verbalize) the specific occurrence and then thank the customer for their patience.

In my experience, I have found that an apology for running behind is an important initial step. Often this can be followed by a sincere thank you for their patience. Finally, the medical professional should sit down, look relaxed and composed (not rushed or flustered), and give the visit the appropriate time it deserves.

Interestingly, some patients understand the situation, appreciate the process, and make efforts to be more direct and to the point.

Patient does not believe diagnosis—Diffuse the situation by personally stating that it sure looks like the condition the NP or PA feels it is, and follow this by stating, "If you can allow us to try this treatment for a few weeks, we can test the treatment for the condition it looks most like."

This first phase can be followed by something like the following, if necessary. "Now, I have been wrong and will continue to be in the future, but we have handled many cases like yours. A biopsy can be performed and will sometimes yield helpful information. (If it looks like a biopsy is not necessary, one can add that, at this time, it might not give us as much information as we would like, so if we can try the treatment for X weeks, we can see if the condition improves). If you would prefer, we can have a review by ___ (the NP or PA can offer appointment with dermatologist)."

This process provides the patient an opportunity to choose. Once they are given an opportunity to participate in the care, they often feel more involved and trusting.

Obviously there are variables, and the situation must be judged on a case-by-case basis, but having a discussion with your NP or PA about options before such a situation occurs can give them a reference point to handle varied situations.

Complicated case that needs joint care (when NP or PA feels under the level of skill or training)—I can see the patient in clinic right away with them.

I use this method the first one to two years in our training of the NP or PA. If they have more experience and do not routinely need the help, I have also told them to schedule a challenging patient at the end of the day on both of our schedules. This works well at educating the NP or PA and letting the patient know we work as a team. The method is also useful when a patient may need a more rapid follow-up than my schedule might allow.

Here are some additional solutions that may work well for the NP or PA.

Ask the patient questions. Asking questions and then allowing time for a response can provide valuable information.

If a patient appears agitated, let them know you sense they may be agitated or frustrated. From here is okay to state, "I sense you are frustrated. Do you mind if I ask if you are?" If the answer is yes, follow up with, "Why are you frustrated?" It is important here not to take offense to what the patient states but rather let them talk. Simply acknowledge their frustration and let them speak.

In the previous scenario, and others I have found, asking questions can be powerful since it allows the patient an opportunity to participate and communicate. At times, the patient needs more of a voice in the situation or their care.

Grant them access when their temper flares. Some are frustrated after waiting a few weeks to see a primary physician or urgent care provider, who then referred them to dermatology. Then the patient had to wait additional days to see the NP or PA. And then the NP or PA tells them something they do not want to hear.

When this happens, give the patient a way to get access to a rapid appointment with the dermatologist. In our practice, we put a note in the chart and ask the patient to call and speak with a medical assistant, who will review the chart and get the provider involved. Our medical assistants or a provider can then overbook the patient or put in for a rapid appointment, if necessary.

Let them share their story. Though this is not always possible, many patients feel the need to let you know the backstory.

It is so common that, as I write this today, I just had a patient who was adamant the rash on his hands did not have cause of allergy or anything he could contribute to be the cause. He stated his medications had not changed, his shampoo was the same, his diet was the same. . . . The list went on. He would not let me get a word in edgewise. After he exhausted himself, I was able to describe (though, again, it took a few more pauses) how his skin has changed, the hot tub he uses interacts uniquely with his skin, and the environment had low humidity recently, which contributes. Finally, he allowed me to share his xerotic dermatitis treatment plan and some recommendations to facilitate emollients. After this, he was more inclined to follow a treatment plan.

It has taken years to learn how to handle patients who have a large laundry list, are overly stressed, or are hyperverbal. I profess not to have any specific approach, but can share one more of the techniques I have found helpful.

And that is, to *care*. Things go better if you care. They also go better if the person you are talking to, aka the patient, feels you do care for their success and well-being. Make sure your NP or PA know the patient can feel the presence of a provider who truly wants them better and cares for them as an individual.

Reminding your NP or PA that each patient is a person who either has a problem, a fear, or is seeking counsel from them is important. The role a health care provider takes on is one to be honored and cherished for the good, which can be done for each individual patient, during each encounter, during each day.

We must remind our NP or PA of the importance they play in people's lives one person at a time.

Part Five

Where This Book Came from
and Where to Take This Knowledge

Chapter 53
Systematic Training:
The Origination Story

Years ago, when I first thought about hiring an NP or a PA, I was overwhelmed. I was working eleven to twelve hours a day trying to keep up. It was a wonderful problem to have, but not one I could appreciate so much at the time. After working several years to grow the practice, I was so blessed to be in a position of needing help seeing patients.

There was no place to schedule punch biopsy follow-ups. There were no urgent patient spots or work-in spots, so I just kept adding patients on. The days kept growing longer.

Though compensated well for my time, I felt frazzled and, frankly, overwhelmed.

Somewhere along the way, the thought of hiring an NP or a PA was floated. At first, it was only an idea. I was not quite ready to give up patients. And, living in a smaller community, I knew getting another dermatologist to partner with would be difficult.

Gradually I heard of other physicians who invested three months in training an NP or a PA and then had help, at least on the patients with straightforward diagnoses. This idea grew on me.

After a year or two of considering options to help me get control of my days and meet the needs of the patients, I decided to take the plunge.

What plunge? The hiring of a nurse practitioner. The process turned out to be way more complicated than I could have imagined.

When we started our practice, I had met a nurse practitioner who expressed interest in joining me. At that time, I did not feel that I was busy enough to justify hiring her. A few years later, I was peddling as fast as I could, and she was working for a neurosurgeon spending weekends on call, rounding on patients outside clinic hours, and telling me she felt like she had no life.

Seeing her in the hospital one night when I was doing a consult, I reminded her of our conversation years before about teaming up.

After a few months, this nurse practitioner mentioned she would like to trade in neurosurgery if she could work in dermatology with me. We discussed her joining again, and she accepted. Her reasoning was she wanted an outpatient clinic, her weekends back to herself, and she would love learning a new specialty. She liked education so much that she wanted to get her doctorate in nursing as well.

Back to the plunge—hiring a nurse practitioner. I thought I had the perfect candidate, because she would be so appreciative of the good hours, no weekends, and would be intellectual, as evidenced by her desire for continued education. Unfortunately, *the plunge* was way more challenging than I imagined.

I had given her what I felt was fair.

- I paid a strong base pay with three months of a slight discount built in, which coincided with me giving her educational time during the clinic each week.
- She would have a half day each week to read and learn on the job. The rest of the time she would follow me and help in the clinic.

I soon found out she was inspired by the doctorate of nursing degree and planned to devote outside time to attaining this, even before mastering dermatology. In addition, she stated she was unhappy having to work and study more than forty hours a week.

After the three-month training period, I overheard my staff mention that she was nowhere close to being able to see patients independently, at least with any dermatology proficiency.

On top of her not being competent in dermatology, she began to complain and point the finger at me that she was not being educated well.

In my small town, I did not want word to get out that I was not providing the most outstanding care. Worse was that the practice had a reputation of being one of excellence in diagnosis and management of skin conditions. There was no room for her skills and performance to be subpar.

I had a hard time adjusting to someone who had the mentality of an hourly employee but was taking the role of a health care provider learning a new specialty.

Her continued complaining made me a bit embarrassed, as though it were my fault she was not learning. She became incessantly diligent in her complaints that the education was not what she needed to be competent.

The comments made me uneasy. I began spending time each weekend—and before long found out it took most of my weekends—to create PowerPoints and lectures for this provider. Even though my day job as a dermatologist for my patients was as full as full could be, I pressed on. I began sharing lectures with her. Though I was more exhausted than before she had been hired, there was great satisfaction in knowing others (my patients and referring doctors) would not throw stones at me for not providing the best education for her.

She continued to kayak on the weekends, share stories of her adventures after work hours, and discuss plans to get her doctorate in nursing. But she never could quite get the knowledge to formulate a differential diagnosis, which created a problem of accuracy in patient care.

The situation led me to add more photos to the lectures, utilize differential diagnosis sessions that we would review together, and spend time after clinic reviewing patients with her.

I soon realized the nurse practitioner would not be able to meet the needs of a growing practice, and so I hired a physician assistant. At this point, the lectures, differential diagnosis sessions, and teaching notes became the basis for creating a system of education for the new hire.

The work on this educational training became somewhat of an obsession for me to find what methods and modalities could help nurse practitioners and physician assistants pick up dermatology skills the fastest. I found the techniques, tools, and methods that they seemed to remember easiest. Many of these centered around building a basic foundation of core principles anchored in understanding the differential diagnosis.

The lectures and techniques we experimented with were reworked and refined until I felt I had a system in place that made learning more straight-forward and simple.

After years of working on training methods, which proved to be immensely helpful and successful for the PA, we found we could use these methods and tools again and again.

As the practice grew, portions of the content were also able to be used with rotating family practice residents, with the medical students I taught as the Indiana University Medical School - South Bend Dermatology Clerkship director, and rotating nurse practitioners and physician assistants.

Thus, our practice had developed a system to hire and train providers.

It was from here that the content was shared with a few of my close colleagues in dermatology. The rave reviews led to further development, including alpha and beta test groups, refinements, and improvements.

The end result is the Dermwise Quick Start Online Training System, which is designed to reduce the burden for training by supervising physicians, educate non-dermatologists in the specialty of dermatology, and also to give verification through examinations of knowledge.

If you would like to enhance the quality of education you provide to your NP or PA and have their competency verified by examinations, then Dermwise is designed for you. At the same time, combining some of the integration techniques (biography sheets, new patient letter, etc.) presented in this text and sharing with your patients the investment you have put into your NP or PA through Dermwise can be a major marketing boost.

A great way to solidify your practice is provide the absolute best care and let your patients know you will not settle for anything else. You can then demonstrate this by sharing the education you provide to their NP or PA. You would be amazed at the number of referrals and word-of-mouth advertising you gain.

To learn more, visit www.dermwise.com.

I wish you outstanding, long-lasting success as you continue to grow your dermatology practice.

Chapter 54
Your Tomorrows

It is my firm belief that the realm of health care is moving fast to involve more nurse practitioners and physician assistants in patient care. As a dermatologist, I initially refused to accept these non-dermatologists into our world of skin care. In fact, I stood firmly against this movement. Now I see, that in all likelihood, this shift in care across all medical specialties is inevitable. The successful practices will embrace the change or face the challenge of fighting the giant behemoth that health care is becoming.

It is my firm belief that if this movement for nurse practitioners and physician assistants is inevitable, we as dermatologists must take the steps necessary to not only embrace the change, but raise the bar. What do I mean? The time is now for those who are involved in hiring, educating, and utilizing the nurse practitioner or physician assistant world to make sure the training is the highest level it can be.

In our practice, our new hires are told their knowledge and training is expected to be higher than any primary care provider in the area. Now, that may or may not always happen, since we have some excellent primary care providers where I live, but it is the standard to which they will be held in our office. They are expected in our small town to have a knowledge of dermatology that is second to only the dermatologist. The bar is set high.

The dermatologists can thus take heed to the changes in health care. The content in this book, coupled with the Dermwise Training System, provides the simplest training, education, and validation of knowledge that can take place in this rapidly changing world of medicine. The steps outlined here, coupled with Dermwise, do the heavy lifting for those practices that want to stay relevant in the medical future.

Chapter 55
Success, Peace, and Happiness

Though life is not filled with boxes of roses and celebrations awaiting us every day, it is possible to enjoy your work and your life. I have found bringing on a nurse practitioner or physician assistant who enjoys and has a passion for dermatology is a worthy venture.

To play the role of educator and mentor to the next generation of health care providers, is one of the grandest rewards I have found. This may be, in part, because I believe each person I train, whether they stay with me or move on to another provider, has the ability to positively impact thousands of patients each year.

The old analogy of the ripple effect, where a stone is thrown in the water and the resulting ripple can be seen a far distance away, comes to mind. The time we spend sharing our knowledge is not only about the revenue to the practice, but it is also about the change in the life of a person you may never meet. It is about sharing all of the best you have been taught, throughout your entire medical training, to a person who can reach patients every day for the remainder of their career.

If all the information in this book had been known to me before I hired my first nurse practitioner, I could have saved myself incalculable hours and likely have made a quantum leap in my income (multiplied by many years, I might add). But that is such a small portion of what this book is about.

I encourage you, if you have read this book, whether you hire a nurse practitioner or a physician assistant or you choose not to, to think about the true value of your interaction with your patients, your staff, and your nurse practitioner or physician assistant. If you are a bit more aware of the positive impact you can have on another human's life each day, then we have done something that can make the world a better place.

As I complete this book, I would say that hiring a nurse practitioner or physician assistant is not an easy undertaking, but it is one that I have found gratifying and worthwhile on multiple levels.

In your future, may you find your struggles as opportunities for growth, your successes as opportunities to share and be humble, and your joy to be an opportunity to make a positive impact on those around you.

I wish you, your family, and your dermatology team much success, peace, and happiness.

References

NP Central—A comprehensive synopsis of an NP:
http://www.npcentral.net/

Michigan Center for Nursing—A good article on NP
certification, DNP, etc.:
https://www.michigancenterfornursing.org/news/news-reports-
and-data/what-does-%E2%80%9Cdoctor-nursing-
practice%E2%80%9D-mean-you-

Buppert, Carolyn, NP, JD, DISCLOSURES. "Can Family Nurse
Practitioners Own Practices?" http://www.medscape.com/
viewarticle/749157. September 08, 2011.

Callen, Jeffrey P., MD and Kenneth E. Greer, MD, Amy S.
Paller, MD, Leonard J. Swinyer, MD. *Color Atlas of
Dermatology*. S. B. Saunders Company, 2000.

Elder, David and Rosalie Elenitsas, MD, Adam I. Rubin, MD,
Michael Ioffreda, MD, Bernett Johnson Jr., MD, Jeffrey Miller,
MD, O. Fred Miller III, MD. *Synopsis and Atlas of Lever's
Histopathology of the Skin*. Lippincott Williams and Wilkins,
1999.

Habif, Thomas P., MD. *Clinical Dermatology: A Color Guide to
Diagnosis and Therapy*, 6th ed. Elsevier Inc., 2016.

Rapini, Ronald P. *Practical Dermatopathology*. Elsevier Inc.,
2005.

Rose, Colin. *Accelerated Learning*. Dell Publishing, 1985.

SOURCES

Site for statistics and information on-demand for dermatology services:
http://www.harriswilliams.com/sites/default/files/industry_report
s/dermatology_industry_presentation_aug2013.pdf

About the Author

Dr. Roger T. Moore is a board-certified dermatologist and the director and founder of the dermatology practice DermacenterMD, established in 2004. He provides a broad range of services including skin cancer identification and treatment, Mohs micrographic surgery, general dermatology, and cosmetic rejuvenation through minimally invasive techniques. His patient following includes clients who travel from Michigan, Illinois, and Ohio, as well as Indiana to see him in Elkhart, Indiana.

A leader in skin cancer care and education, Dr. Moore has been a speaker at events in a vast geographic footprint extending from his home state of Indiana to Texas and California. He routinely teaches medical providers in his region as well as medical students through his role as the dermatology clinical director at Indiana University School of Medicine - South Bend. He has also hosted nurse practitioners, physician assistants, and resident physicians for rotations through his clinic. He has contributed to research in medical dermatology and in cosmetic procedures, including botulinum toxin.

Dr. Moore knows the importance of continuing his own education. He maintains the highest level of continuing education, including courses from international leaders in cosmetic, medical, and surgical dermatology. He is a diplomate of the American Board of Dermatology, a fellow of the renowned American Academy of Dermatology, American Society of Dermatologic Surgery, American Society for Mohs Micrographic Surgery, and is a member of American Medical Association and Indiana State Medical Association. He takes very seriously his own knowledge and the trust his patients place in him as their provider.